Environmental Health Policy

Understanding Public Health

Series editors: Nick Black and Rosalind Raine, London School of Hygiene & Tropical Medicine

Throughout the world, recognition of the importance of public health to sustainable, safe and healthy societies is growing. The achievements of public health in nineteenth-century Europe were for much of the twentieth century overshadowed by advances in personal care, in particular in hospital care. Now, with the dawning of a new century, there is increasing understanding of the inevitable limits of individual health care and of the need to complement such services with effective public health strategies. Major improvements in people's health will come from controlling communicable diseases, eradicating environmental hazards, improving people's diets and enhancing the availability and quality of effective health care. To achieve this, every country needs a cadre of knowledgeable public health practitioners with social, political and organizational skills to lead and bring about changes at international, national and local levels.

This is one of a series of 20 books that provides a foundation for those wishing to join in and contribute to the twenty-first-century regeneration of public health, helping to put the concerns and perspectives of public health at the heart of policy-making and service provision. While each book stands alone, together they provide a comprehensive account of the three main aims of public health: protecting the public from environmental hazards, improving the health of the public and ensuring high quality health services are available to all. Some of the books focus on methods, others on key topics. They have been written by staff at the London School of Hygiene & Tropical Medicine with considerable experience of teaching public health to students from low, middle and high income countries. Much of the material has been developed and tested with postgraduate students both in face-to-face teaching and through distance learning.

The books are designed for self-directed learning. Each chapter has explicit learning objectives, key terms are highlighted and the text contains many activities to enable the reader to test their own understanding of the ideas and material covered. Written in a clear and accessible style, the series will be essential reading for students taking postgraduate courses in public health and will also be of interest to public health practitioners and policy-makers.

Titles in the series

Analytical models for decision making: Colin Sanderson and Reinhold Gruen
Controlling communicable disease: Norman Noah
Economic analysis for management and policy: Stephen Jan, Lilani Kumaranayake, Jenny Roberts, Kara Hanson and Kate Archibald
Economic evaluation: Julia Fox-Rushby and John Cairns (eds)
Environmental epidemiology: Paul Wilkinson (ed)
Environment, health and sustainable development: Megan Landon
Environmental health policy: David Ball
Financial management in health services: Reinhold Gruen and Anne Howarth
Global change and health: Kelley Lee and Jeff Collin (eds)
Health care evaluation: Sarah Smith, Don Sinclair, Rosalind Raine and Barnaby Reeves
Health promotion practice: Wendy Macdowall, Chris Bonell and Maggie Davies (eds)
Health promotion theory: Maggie Davies and Wendy Macdowall (eds)
Introduction to epidemiology: Lucianne Bailey, Katerina Vardulaki, Julia Langham and Daniel Chandramohan
Introduction to health economics: David Wonderling, Reinhold Gruen and Nick Black
Issues in public health: Joceline Pomerleau and Martin McKee (eds)
Making health policy: Kent Buse, Nicholas Mays and Gill Walt
Managing health services: Nick Goodwin, Reinhold Gruen and Valerie Iles
Medical anthropology: Robert Pool and Wenzel Geissler
Principles of social research: Judith Green and John Browne (eds)
Understanding health services: Nick Black and Reinhold Gruen

Environmental Health Policy

David Ball

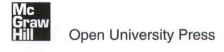
Open University Press

Open University Press
McGraw-Hill Education
McGraw-Hill House
Shoppenhangers Road
Maidenhead
Berkshire
England
SL6 2QL

email:enquiries@openup.co.uk
world wide web: www.openup.co.uk

and Two Penn Plaza, New York, NY 10121-2289, USA

First published 2006

A catalogue record of this book is available from the British Library

ISBN-10: 0 335 21843 1 (pb)
ISBN-13: 978 0 335 21843 1 (pb)

Library of Congress Cataloging-in-Publication Data
CIP data applied for

Typeset by RefineCatch Limited, Bungay, Suffolk
Printed in the UK by Bell & Bain Ltd, Glasgow

The **McGraw·Hill** Companies

Contents

Acknowledgements

Open University Press and the London School of Hygiene & Tropical Medicine have made every effort to obtain permission from copyright holders to reproduce material in this book and to acknowledge these sources correctly. Any omissions brought to our attention will be remedied in future editions.

We would like to express our grateful thanks to the following copyright holders for granting permission to reproduce material in this book.

Chapter 1

Table 1.1 from IRGC (2005).

Chapter 2

Extracts from Covello and Mumpower (1985: 4, 8, 9).

Chapter 3

Figure 3.1 from Ball (2000); Figure 3.2 from NRC Red Book (1983); Table 3.1 from BMA (1987); extract from NRC Red Book (1983: 4–5).

Chapter 4

Extract from Ottoboni (1991: 26, 27); extract from Commonwealth of Australia (2002: 52–3).

Chapter 5

Extracts from Paustenbach (1989: 82–3, 86–7, 87–9); extract from Commonwealth of Australia (2002: 78–80).

Chapter 6

Extracts from Covello and Merkhofer (1993: 92–4, 117); extract from Rodricks (1992: 16–17); Figure 6.5 from Rodricks (1992: 28).

Chapter 7

Extract from Paustenbach (1989: 90–1); Table 7.1 from Rodricks (1992: 188–9); Figure 7.1 from HMSO (1995); Figures 7.2 and 7.3 from HMSO (1989).

Chapter 8

Table 8.1 from *Environment International* 28 (2002); Figure 8.1 from *The Green Book* (2003); Figure 8.3 from Ball DJ and Soby B (1995) Valuing consumer safety. *International Journal for Consumer Safety* 2(3): 171–131. Taylor & Francis Ltd, http://www.tandf.co.uk/journals; Figure 8.4 from *Accident Analysis and Prevention* 32 (2000); extract from *Risk Analysis* 25(4) (2005).

Chapter 9

Figures 9.1, 9.2 and 9.3 from UNEP (1985); extract from UNEP (1985); extract and Figure 9.5 from Stokell et al. (1991); Figure 9.4 from NRPB slide pack; extract and Figure 9.6 from Ball DJ and Goats GC (1996) Risk management and consumer safety. *International Journal for Consumer Safety* 3(3): 111–124. Taylor & Francis Ltd, http://www.tandf.co.uk/journals; Figure 9.7 from ISOE.

Chapter 10

Extract from WHO (1987); Figure 10.2 from HMSO (1988); extract from Ball DJ and Goats GC (1996) Risk management and consumer safety. *International Journal for Consumer Safety* 3(3): 111–124. Taylor & Francis Ltd, http://www.tandf.co.uk/journals; extracts from Kocher (1996); Figure 10.3 from MCA (2006); extract and Figures 10.4 and 10.5 from Travis et al. (1987).

Chapter 11

Extracts from Schwartz and Thompson (1990: 17), *Human and Ecological Risk Assessment.* 6(4) (2000), and Arrow et al. (1996).

Chapter 12

Figure 12.1 from www.asiantsunamivideos.com/; Figure 12.2 from Lichtenstein et al. (1978); Figures 12.3, 12.4 and 12.5 from Slovic (2000: 114, 99, 142); Figure 12.6 from Eiser (2004: 40); Table 12.1 from Eiser (2004: 20).

Chapter 13

Extract from Adams (1995: 34); extract from Schwartz and Thompson (1990: 6); extract from Adams and Thompson (2002: 18–22); Figures 13.1, 13.2, 13.3 and 13.4 from Adams (1995: 34, 35, 36, 202).

Chapter 14

Figures 14.1, 14.2 and 14.3 from BMA (1998: 36, 51 and 82); extracts from Thérivel and Partidário (1996: 4–5, 104–8); extracts from Joyce (2001: 8, 9–10).

Chapter 15

Table 15.1 from Ames et al. (1987); extract from Strategic Advisory Board (1990); Tables 15.3 and 15.4 from US Strategic Advisory Board (1990); extract from Clarence-Davies (1996: 78, 79).

Chapter 16

Extracts from O'Brien (2000: 120–1, xiii–xiv, 131–2, 133–4, 143–5); extract from Sunstein (2002: 102–4).

Chapter 17

Table 17.1 from *Risk Analysis* 15(2) (1995); Figures 17.2 and 17.3 and extract from IRGC (2005: 53, 13, 15); Figure 17.1 from NRC (1996: 28); extract from NRC (1996: 22–3); Figure 17.4 from Lundgren (1994: 3); Figure 17.5 from *Risk Analysis* 23(5) (2003); extracts from Löfstedt (2005; 19, 21).

Chapter 18

Extracts from Seedhouse (2000: 53–6, 77–8); Figure 18.1 © Ortwin Renn (2005); extract from Graham (2001); extract from Lichtenstein et al. (1990).

Chapter 19

Extracts from UNDP (2006); extract from Kiyn (2006); Figure 19.1 and extract from Coggan et al. (2000); extract from Nilsen (2004); Activity 19.4 is based on Seedhouse (1997).

Chapter 20

Extracts and Table 20.1 from Graham and Wiener (1995); extract from Bial et al. (2000); extract from O'Brien (2000).

Overview of the book

Introduction

The issue of environmental health policy occupies a prominent position on both local and global agendas as old and new challenges confront the human race. There is a continual requirement for policies that will deal effectively with a seemingly never-ending supply of hazards that impinge on health and well-being. The challenge faced by policy makers is by no means straightforward. Policies must not only be effective, they must also be efficient in their use of resources, for there are never enough resources to go around. In addition, policies generally need the support of the people for whom they are designed if they are to work, so not only is it necessary to understand policy issues objectively, there is also a subjective element which needs to be taken into account.

For this reason, no single discipline could possibly provide a full description of the roots and mechanisms of environmental health policy. This book, therefore, sets out to provide a multidisciplinary window onto environmental policy and its formulation. From this you will observe both the order that exists at the centre, and the controversies around the borders. Since there is no such thing as a recipe for making policy, every circumstance being unique, policy makers are best equipped for the task if they fully understand the nature of the task, the tools at their disposal and the likely complexities of the situations to be encountered.

Many of the themes raised in this book have been developed in companion volumes in the series, often from a different perspective. To view things from different perspectives is useful for a deeper understanding even if the accounts are not entirely consistent. This book explores the roots of many controversies without necessarily providing answers. What it will do is increase your insight and hence ability to make those difficult choices demanded of anyone contributing to environmental health policy.

It is accepted that you already will have your own views on environmental health and related policies based on your own professional background and experience. This will provide an interesting backcloth against which to work through the book. However, because of the multidisciplinary approach, some of the material may be very new, but no specialist knowledge is required. At the end, you should be in a stronger position to interpret the complex technical and social issues surrounding environmental health policy and be better equipped to form your own perspective on them.

Why study environmental health policy?

Before beginning, let us ask why would you, or anyone, want to study environmental health policy and what might be the benefits if you did? Listed here are some reasons, though you might well be able to think of others, either now or later:

1 It might not always be obvious, but environmental health policies, even their absence, affect us all.
2 Health and the environment are of great importance to most people.
3 The world faces major environmental health challenges at the local, regional and global level.
4 Environmental health policies require and consume vast resources. There are never enough resources to go around, so it is important to try to make the best use of them.
5 Where environmental health policy is affecting people's health and welfare, those people will be more enfranchised if they understand the different ways in which policy is formed.
6 If you aspire to work in the policy field, it is essential that you understand the bases of policy, including the strengths and limitations of different approaches to policy formulation, in order to do the best job.
7 There are many forces affecting the evolution of policy, some intentionally and some inadvertently. If good policy decisions are to be made, these forces need to be recognized and understood.
8 The indirect implications of environmental health policies on lifestyles, communities and businesses are also significant. This needs to be observed and considered.

Structure of the book

This book is based on the conceptual outline of the 'Environmental Health Policy' unit taught at the London School of Hygiene & Tropical Medicine. It was reviewed, and updated in 2005–6, and adapted for distance learning.

The book traces an evolving story, focusing on the past 20 years of development right up to the present. The policy-making process continues to adjust, so being aware of changes of emphasis, and the reasons for them, strengthens understanding. Understanding is paramount if you are to implement effective policy. The approach draws on the natural and biological sciences, economics, sociology, psychology, communication, philosophy and politics. Do not be put off by this – all is explained.

The book is comprised of seven sections and 20 chapters. Each chapter is set out in this way:

• an overview
• a list of learning objectives
• a list of key terms
• a range of activities
• feedback on the activities
• a summary.

All chapters have references, some of which you might want to follow up, though the text is self-contained. A great deal of useful material can also be found on the internet.

Although examples and case studies in this book are drawn from low, middle and high income countries, you should be aware that most of the theory on environmental health policy which is used internationally, has originated in English-speaking, mainly higher income countries, and has spread around the world through its use by international agencies, both public and private. Policy making of the type described here also tends to be practised more at the level of central and regional government, though this should not deter others from seeking an understanding of the procedure, as everyone is a part of the system and knowledge assists enfranchisement.

The description of the section and chapter contents will give you an idea of what will follow.

Section 1, Introduction. Chapter 1 asks what is meant by 'environmental health' and 'environmental health policy'. It points out choices which can be made regarding the former, and, by way of an analysis of some general principles of environmental health policy, identifies the key factors on the minds of most environmental policy makers at the start of the twenty-first century. The chapter concludes by noting that an impressive array of tools have been devised to help policy makers. Chapter 2 explores the background to one of these tools (others come later) which has achieved notable prominence internationally, namely, health risk assessment. How has it come about and why is it important now?

Section 2, Assessing environmental health risks. Chapters 3–7 constitute the main scientific input to the book. Even for non-scientists with an interest in environmental health policy, it is important to have an idea of where the scientific knowledge comes from and on what basis. Without that, you would not be able to assess its merits and ask questions. Chapter 3 gives an overview of the now dominant model of health risk assessment, breaking it down into its component stages. Chapters 4–7 take you through each of these stages, giving you solid grounding from which to move on to other topics.

Section 3, Rational action and environmental health policy. In this third section you will move on from assessing risks to the various models that can help you decide, once you have assessed them, what should be done. Should a risk be tolerated, and if not, by how much should it be reduced? As a first step to answering this question, Chapter 8 considers the contribution of economics to environmental decision making. Building upon this, Chapters 9 and 10 then examine national and international frameworks for decision making involving hazards of three kinds: environmental, radiological, and safety. From this emerges a 'rational' model of policy making, grounded in science and economics.

Section 4, Beyond the rational action approach. There is no avoiding the fact that environmental health policy decisions are frequently controversial, and it would be pointless to pretend otherwise. Indeed, the 'rational' model described in the previous section does not find universal acceptance. To this end, Section 4 introduces some very different ideas about how decisions are and should be made so that the reasons for these disputes over policy can be understood. Chapter 11 describes arguments (and counter-arguments) that are lodged against the scientific and economic approaches to policy formulation. It also gives an overview of competing theories that offer alternative views. One of these, described in Chapter 12, is the psychometric paradigm. This is about how risks are perceived, rather than how they actually are. An understanding of the public perception of risks is essential for most present-day policy makers. Chapter 13 introduces one more sociological theory, cultural theory, which takes a very different line on how controversies arise and what to do about them. It has important advice to offer policy makers, as well as providing an illuminating view of the nature of policy arguments.

Section 5, Other approaches. If the rational model of decision making is challenged, what else is there? The three chapters in this section take you through a range of alternatives, including environmental impact assessment, health impact assessment, social impact assessment, strategic environmental assessment, environmental risk ranking, alternatives assessment and the precautionary principle. The emphasis is not on providing a detailed account, for this is done well in other books, but on asking why these alternatives are forthcoming and what it is that they offer which is new.

Section 6, Making policy. By now it will be plain, if it was not before, that modern environmental health policy making is not only about 'science' but also about communication and people's values. Chapter 17 is about why communication is important, how it can be an integral part of the policy process, and the style of communication that is appropriate. Underlying everything, though, is philosophy and politics. Chapter 18 returns head-on to the issue of controversy in policy making and examines, from these perspectives, why it can be so divisive. This is not so that it can be made argument-free, but so that the nature of arguments can be understood. From that vantage point policy makers, for whom 'The buck stops here', are hopefully better equipped to do their jobs.

Section 7, Initiatives – local to global. Section 7 analyses some current environmental health policy initiatives. Chapter 19 focuses on 'local' initiatives such as Agenda 21, Capacity 21, and various interventions aimed at creating healthier communities. What lies behind them, what makes them 'tick', are they effective and what is the evidence? Chapter 20 switches to the complexities of global environmental programmes designed to deal with stratospheric ozone depletion and greenhouse gas emissions. Why does the resolution of environmental health issues at the global level present such an apparently intractable problem? What, realistically, can be achieved?

A variety of activities are included to help you understand and assimilate the topics and ideas presented. These include:

- questions based on reading influential articles from books and research papers;
- analysis of quantitative and qualitative data;
- reflection involving your own knowledge, experience and circumstances.

The author acknowledges and thanks Megan Landon who developed the original course at the LSHTM and who thus provided the broad outline for the book, and also for several of the case studies. Thanks are also due to Professor Nick Black for reviewing the text and to Avril Porter for managing its production.

SECTION 1

Introduction

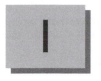

Introduction to environmental health policy

Overview

In this introductory chapter you will first consider several definitions of 'environmental health'. It will help to clarify which definition is relevant to your own interests, though it is possible that this may change as you progress. Whatever your personal interest, however, it is important that you are aware of the different interpretations that others might legitimately place on this term, since you will certainly encounter them. Second, you will examine the array of principles that impact upon environmental health policy as currently practised. Finally, you will receive a brief and preliminary introduction to the key tools recommended by international agencies, governments and other organizations as aids for decision makers in determining their policies.

Learning objectives

By the end of this chapter, you will be better able to:

- **identify different interpretations of environmental health**
- **specify your own environmental health interests while acknowledging those of other people**
- **list considerations that typically influence the formulation of environmental health policy**
- **name some of the principal tools used in environmental health assessment.**

Key terms

Environmental health Those aspects of human health and disease that are determined by factors in the environment.

Policy Broad statement of goals, objectives and means that create the framework for activity. Often taking the form of explicit written documents but may also be implicit or unwritten.

What is environmental health?

Before studying environmental health policy, you need to consider what is meant by the term 'environmental health' and what it means to you or your organization. One definition can be found in the European Charter, *Environment and Health*

(WHO 1990). According to this, environmental health comprises *those aspects of human health and disease that are determined by factors in the environment.* The European Charter also says that the term refers to the *theory and practice of assessing and controlling* factors in the environment that can potentially affect health.

However, this definition is still open to interpretation. For example, for some agencies, environmental health is primarily associated with the direct pathological effects of 'chemicals, radiation and some biological agents' whereas others additionally include 'the effects (often indirect) of the broad physical, social and aesthetic environment, which includes housing, urban development, land use and transport' (WHO 1990).

Many agencies, including the WHO, are also concerned about the impact upon health and safety attributable to injuries. Injuries themselves may arise from contact with either the natural or the man-made environment. Or they may be accidental, self-inflicted or associated with some malicious act. When thinking about environmental health policy it is necessary to decide which, if any, of these additional issues fall within your domain of interest.

There is a further definitional issue. In talking about environmental health, many groups are concerned primarily or solely with risks to people. Their goal is the preservation of human life and the improvement of human health. However, there are others who are at least as much concerned or possibly more so with the non-human, but living environment, and yet others still who are concerned with the non-living environment, for example, the rocks beneath our feet, irrespective of whether there are any living organisms around to enjoy them. It can, of course, be argued that, because human beings are part of the wider ecosystem, a healthy environment is necessary to maintain human health. It could also be argued that humans have a moral duty, whether it benefits them directly or not, to look after the environment for the sake of other living organisms, or even to look after it simply because it is there. Table 1.1 is a list of risks that might be incorporated under the heading of 'environmental health'.

 Activity 1.1

Examine Table 1.1 and, thinking about where you live and your own interests, answer the following questions:

1 What aspects of environmental health do you consider should be included in your working definition, and why?
2 Are there any persons or groups in the place in which you live or work who might favour a different definition and, if so, why?

 Feedback

Basically, it is a matter of choice as to which definition of environmental health you select. There is no 'correct' answer. Table 1.1 shows how wide the possibilities can be. Whatever you decide, it is important to be aware of where you draw the boundaries and also why other people might draw them differently.

Table 1.1 A taxonomy of risk types according to hazardous agents

Hazardous agents	Risk
Physical agents	Ionizing radiation
	Non-ionizing radiation
	Noise
	Kinetic energy (explosion, collapse, etc.)
	Temperature (fire, overheating, cold)
	Physical hazards (unsafe premises, public spaces, etc.)
Chemical agents	Toxic substances (with thresholds)
	Genotoxic/carcinogenic substances
	Environmental pollutants
	Mixtures
Biological agents	Fungi and algae
	Bacteria
	Viruses
	Genetically modified organisms
	Other pathogens
Natural forces	Wind
	Earthquakes
	Volcanic activities
	Mudslides
	Drought
	Floods
	Tsunamis
	Bush fires
	Avalanches
Socio-communicative hazards	Human violence (criminal acts)
	Humiliation, mobbing
	Terrorism and sabotage
	Mass hysteria
	Psychosomatic syndromes
Complex hazards (combinations)	Food (chemical and biological hazards)
	Consumer products (chemical, physical etc. characteristics)
	Technologies (physical, chemical, etc.)
	Large constructions (buildings, dams, highways, bridges, etc.)
	Critical infrastructures (physical, economic, social/organizational and communicative)

Source: Adapted from IRGC (2005)

Environmental health policy

A policy is defined as 'a course or principle of action adopted or proposed by a government, party, business, or individual etc.' (*Concise Oxford Dictionary* 1991). Policies are normally based on a set of underlying principles. These principles must be related to the issue of concern, in this case, environmental health. In other literature you might also come across the terms 'plan', and 'programme'. The difference between policies, plans and programmes is not clearly defined, but a fairly common explanation might be: 'A policy may . . . be considered as the inspiration and guidance for action, a plan as a set of coordinated and timed objectives for the implementation of the policy, and a programme as a set of projects in a particular area' (Wood and Djeddour 1992).

 Activity 1.2

Thinking about your own situation, write down some underlying principles that might help you develop a strategic policy on environmental health. This is quite a difficult question at this stage if you are new to this field, so do not be concerned if you find it hard. Later, it will become much easier.

 Feedback

Many organizations list their guiding principles on the world-wide web. For example, on its website: www.cieh.org, the London-based Chartered Institute of Environmental Health (CIEH) lists its principles as:

- concerns for human health and well-being, and the desire to improve this through appropriate environmental change and intervention;
- equity, and the wish to promote the benefits of the environmental health approach to all members and sections of society including the most disadvantaged;
- precaution, because it is believed that prevention of harm is better than cure;
- an holistic approach, because of the linkage between environmental, social and economic factors and their collective impact upon health and well-being;
- sustainability, in recognition of the need to create and maintain future conditions which will secure health and well-being;
- civic participation, because of the requirement that environmental health policy recognize the role of public concerns and the need to maintain openness and transparency in decision-making processes;
- recognition of the forces of globalization, and the fact that environmental health problems do not respect man-made borders.

Factors bearing upon environmental health policy

The above principles adopted by the CIEH are of special interest because they refer to many considerations which are on the minds of present-day environmental health policy makers.

 Activity 1.3

Read through the CIEH principles carefully and make a note of those words and phrases which you think might be important to policy makers.

Feedback

You might have noted the following features of the principles. Do not be concerned if you did not identify all or even many of them, as you now are only at the point where the stage is being set. Nonetheless, it will help you, as you progress, to be able to link sections of this book to sets of principles such as these. What might at first seem like disparate topics will more easily be seen to belong to a whole.

The first principle refers to both health *and* welfare, a theme also picked up by the World Health Organization (WHO) in its writings. The implication is that the interest is not only in the absence of disease, illness and injury, but also wider issues of social welfare and fulfilment. More subtly, the first principle also uses the word 'appropriate' when talking about environmental change and intervention. The matter of what is an 'appropriate' change or intervention is of deep significance to policy makers, as you will discover as you progress through this book.

The second principle raises the issue of 'equity'. Equity considerations are now higher on the agenda of policy makers than previously. As you read on, you will understand how this situation arose and the arguments around it. Likewise, the third principle raises an entirely different principle of 'precaution'. It is probable that you have heard of the 'precautionary principle', and this alludes to it. Policy makers need to understand what this principle is, and when and how to apply it.

The fourth principle introduces the idea of an 'holistic approach', one which is said to recognize the link between environmental, social and economic factors in affecting health. This, as you will discover, marks another important shift which has occurred in thinking in environmental health policy making, and has resulted in the development of many new tools to aid policy makers. The fifth principle brings in yet another concept of great influence in modern policy making, that of 'sustainability'.

The sixth principle ventures onto more new ground, that of civic participation in environmental health policy and the need to recognize public concerns and be accountable and transparent. This is why environmental health policy makers need to be familiar with the psychology of risk perception, and methods of risk communication and deliberation. The final principle points out that environmental health issues are not confined to the local, but have regional and even global dimensions.

By the time you have finished this book, you will have studied every one of these items and have much to say about them. Their commonality, through sets of principles like these, is worth keeping in mind.

Policy tools

The above principles of the CIEH contain all the essential elements with which present-day policy makers are likely to be concerned. Other agencies will use different words, but the essence will be basically the same. To help policy makers address these elements, many tools have been devised. You may already be aware, or if not, will soon observe, that great emphasis is seen to have been placed upon the use of *risk assessment* in particular, in documents published by agencies such as the World Health Organization and the United Nations (UN). For example,

Agenda 21, which was designed by the UN as a comprehensive plan of global action aimed at integrating environmental and development issues, including health, into decision making (see Chapter 19), makes extensive reference to the use of risk assessment in determining action plans. Risk-based thinking, of which risk assessment is a part, has, in fact, become an almost standard approach to decision making and can be found in all countries of the world, particularly in national and regional agencies, but is gradually spreading downwards to the local level. Because of its importance, this book continues with a detailed description of the techniques associated with this approach, before moving on to examine other techniques including environmental impact assessment, health impact assessment, and social impact assessment, which have been devised, sometimes in response to perceived weaknesses in risk-based approaches, and at other times to complement them.

As a further indication of what lies ahead, Table 1.2 sets out a fairly typical view of the necessary components of an environmental management framework. Although based on a manufacturing company's view of its responsibilities, general environmental emphases are present. As you can see, under the human and environmental safety element, the key tools identified are human health risk assessment, which is the main concern here, and ecological risk assessment. However, other entries are pertinent to our interest, including the efficient use of resources, and hence economic analysis, and addressing what are described as 'societal concerns'. This brings in tools related to 'understanding' and 'responding',

Table 1.2 An overall framework for environmental management of a manufacturing facility

Goal	Elements	Key tools
	Human and environmental safety	Human health risk assessment Ecological risk assessment
	Regulatory compliance	Site auditing Waste reporting Material consumption reporting New chemicals testing Product classification and labelling
Environmentally and economically sustainable environmental management	Efficient use of resources and waste management	Waste and energy monitoring Material use monitoring Environmental auditing of site Supplier auditing Product life cycle analysis Economic analysis
	Addressing societal concerns	Understanding: • opinion surveys • consumer research • dialogue Responding through: • public presentations and publications • working groups • reporting • cooperation with society to find solutions to environmental problems

Source: Adapted from White et al. (1995)

all of which ties in with the guiding principles of the CIEH and other agencies working in the field of environmental health policy.

Summary

In this introductory chapter you thought about the scope of your interests regarding environmental health and noted that others might legitimately define their interests in another way. You examined a typical set of principles of an agency whose interest is environmental health policy, and noted how these principles are concerned with a host of issues ranging from health (of course), to welfare, appropriateness of interventions, equity, precaution, holism, sustainability, participation and globalization. The promise has been made that all these will be covered in this book. Finally, you are aware of the existence of an array of tools which have been devised to help environmental health policy makers perform their duties, and which will be described in later chapters.

References

International Risk Governance Council (2005) *Risk Governance: Towards an Integrative Approach*. Geneva: IRGC.

White PR, De Smet B, Owens JW and Hindel P (1995) Environmental management in an international consumer goods company. *Resources, Conservation and Recycling* 14(1): 171–84.

Wood C and Djeddour M (1992) Strategic environmental assessment: environmental assessment of policies, plans and programmes. *The Impact Assessment Bulletin* 10(1): 3–22.

World Health Organization Regional Office for Europe (1990) *Environment and Health: The European Charter and Commentary*. WHO Regional Publications, European Series No. 35. Copenhagen: WHO Regional Office.

2 The emergence of risk assessment

Overview

In the introductory chapter you learned that a range of tools have been devised to help environmental health policy makers. Paramount among these is risk assessment which is now a major environmental health policy tool used at the local, national and international level as an aid for setting priorities. It is in operation in many other sectors besides environmental health, and this has assisted its rise to prominence. Although risk-based decision making has existed in some form for millennia, the extent of its present-day application is unique. This chapter describes influences affecting the development of risk assessment as an approach to decision making and why its current status is so high. It concludes by examining how the circumstances of risk assessment today differ from those of the past, and by considering the range of applications within environmental health.

Learning objectives

By the end of this chapter, you will be better able to:

- **outline the origins and development of risk-based approaches**
- **identify reasons why risk-based thinking has come to such prominence**
- **discuss emerging factors that influence the way in which risk assessment is conducted**
- **give examples of areas of application.**

Key terms

Probability A quantitative or qualitative expression of the likelihood or chance that a particular outcome will occur as a result of a specified cause or action.

Risk assessment A method for estimating the probability or likelihood of a specified type of harm occurring to an individual or a population.

Risk-based thinking An approach to decision making that relies in part upon risk assessment.

Risk assessment in modern society

The origins of risk assessment can be traced back thousands of years, but it is only in modern times that it has become so highly formalized and the dominant tool in the identification, characterization, and management of health hazards. The approach has been developed simultaneously in many disciplines including epidemiology, toxicology, engineering, mathematics, occupational and public safety, injury prevention, insurance, psychology, sociology and law. Risk assessment is now so deeply embedded in society that risk issues and risk-related ways of thinking are constantly reported in the media around the world. Certainly, in the Western and English-speaking world, it is the dominant paradigm.

 Activity 2.1

Thinking about the country in which you live:

1 Which risks are of current concern?
2 Are these risks the same as those reported in the media?

 Feedback

The answer to these questions will depend very much on the level of industrialization and the culture in which you live.

1 In some high income countries, current preoccupations include risks associated with the use of mobile phones and their associated transmitting stations, genetically modified crops, air pollution, global warming, food additives and lack of exercise. In low and middle income countries concerns may well focus on the risk of natural disasters, the supply and safety of water, the presence of disease, and the occurrence of injuries.

2 These issues attract a great deal of media attention, but this is not necessarily because they pose the greatest threat. While the media often reflect public concern, they have their own interests which may lead to a different perspective being presented from that which is of concern within the population.

Early origins and development of risk-based thinking

There is benefit to be gained in understanding, even briefly, the historical development of this field. This is because the way that activities such as these are conducted and interpreted is never static and an awareness of their past aids understanding of their present and possible future form. To this end, the policy and public affairs experts Vincent Covello and Jeryl Mumpower (1985) have produced an insightful history of risk analysis focusing primarily on the time before the twentieth century. In their work they refer to the existence of simplified forms of risk assessment which were being carried out as long ago as 3200 BC in the Tigris–Euphrates valley and there are almost certainly earlier examples from elsewhere.

However, it was not until the seventeenth and eighteenth centuries that mathematical probability theory and the laws of chance became established, allowing rapid progress. This happened through the work of renowned mathematicians and scientists such as Pascal, Halley, LaPlace and Poisson. As a result of their work, the idea was firmly established that the probability or likelihood of future events could be calculated, a logic which in fact had previously been denied or even discouraged. For example, in 1792, LaPlace made an analysis of the probability of death with and without smallpox vaccination.

However, the question as to why it took so long for probability theory to emerge is not easy to answer. Covello and Mumpower provide several plausible explanations. These include the requirements of the then developing commercial organizations, particularly those dealing with shipping and life insurance, and limitations in mathematical techniques, but they conclude that none of these alone is convincing and point instead to an intriguing argument offered by David (1962) and others, revolving around the attitude of the Christian Church. According to David '[there] seems to have been a taboo on speculations with regard to health, philosophers implying that to count the sick or even the number of boys born was impious in that it probed the inscrutable purpose of God'. Likewise, Grier (1980) argues that much of the intellectual thinking about probability in the seventeenth and eighteenth centuries was rooted in intense discussions in church debates over the morality of charging interest on loans. Risk as a topic was caught up in these ecclesiastical debates because one argument in favour of permitting interest to be charged on loans was that the lender was taking a risk that his money might be lost. This clerical matter, it seemed, needed to be resolved before risk could become a legitimate subject for public discussion. It should be recalled that the penalties of going against the doctrines of the Church could be, in those days, severe.

The development of risk-based thinking was also delayed by another factor. This was the quest for causal links between adverse health effects and different types of hazard (Covello and Mumpower 1985). The main methods of establishing causal links had, throughout history, been based on observation, either involving personal trial and error as in tasting a new fruit, or in observing the effect upon others, including animals, of different diets. On a more sophisticated level, the precursors of modern epidemiological methods which seek to establish associations or cause–effect relationships by the observation of adverse health effects in groups, can be traced back thousands of years to the eras of the Greeks and the Romans, but it was only in the sixteenth to the eighteenth centuries that extensive progress was made. This delay has been attributed to a lack of models of scientific, biological, chemical and physical processes. However, at that time, there were major intellectual developments underway in Europe during the period known as the Enlightenment. Exponents of the Enlightenment believed that human reason could be used to combat ignorance and superstition to build a better world. Their principal targets were the beliefs of the established Church and the domination of society by a hereditary aristocracy. For example, prior to this period, it was believed that most illnesses, injuries, misfortunes and disasters could best be explained in social, religious or magical terms. These views were entrenched and resistant to change.

✎ Activity 2.2

Having read this summary of the historical analysis by Vince Covello and Jeryl Mumpower, write down a list of factors that slowed the emergence of risk-based methods.

Feedback

The potential barriers include limitations of mathematical techniques especially probability theory, lack of demand prior to the emergence of the insurance industry, the limited scientific understanding of the chemical, biological and physical processes which could lead to ill health, and the belief that ill health and injuries were 'punishments from God' and that 'the work of God' should not be a topic of investigation or speculation.

Recent developments

Although, as described above, risk-based thinking is known to have been in use in some form since Babylonian times, its early application was originally restricted mainly to insurance interests, and its application elsewhere, if it existed at all, was less obvious. The insurance industry, nonetheless, had an important role to play in propagating risk-based thinking internationally. In 1688, in London, the first insurance company was formed in Lloyd's coffee house, a place frequented by ship owners, merchants and underwriters, eventually to become one of the first modern insurance companies – Lloyd's of London. As commerce expanded around the world, it was soon realized that insurance presented an important business opportunity and by the late eighteenth century the first companies specializing in fire insurance had been formed in the USA. Other insurance needs were discovered in the coming decades, that of life insurance being one to grow rapidly. Later, the need for 'reinsurance' was identified, by which insured losses were distributed between insurance companies. This realization was prompted by major fires which carried high costs for the insurers. The need for reinsurance is confirmed every time there is a major disaster, as in the 2004 tsunami in the Indian Ocean or the 2005 earthquake in NE Pakistan, or the confirmation of some serious workplace disease such as asbestos-related mesothelioma or lung disease.

Insurance, of course, relies heavily upon actuarial science, that is, the application of statistics to insurance needs. However, the use of statistics didn't stop there. Its use in other sectors developed strongly in the twentieth century. An early application was found in nuclear engineering where issues of rare but potentially catastrophic incidents, as at Chernobyl, had to be considered. As a result, the nuclear industry was influential in taking forward risk-based thinking in the industrial engineering sector, and this momentum was later picked up by other engineering interests such as the offshore oil and gas industry, and the rail, marine and air transport sectors. The international dimension of these activities assisted the rapid spread of the associated thinking to all corners of the globe.

Risk-based thinking was also beginning to manifest itself in important legal cases by the mid-twentieth century and not long after that in national legal statutes and international law. In fact, during the last few decades of the twentieth century, it became a *de facto* requirement in some countries to apply risk-based techniques in fields as diverse as nursing, psychiatry, police work, education, sport and leisure, environmental protection and almost any conceivable human activity. As noted in Chapter 1, UN Agenda 21 also emphasizes the use of risk-based approaches in tackling environmental health hazards, as do many other international programmes.

You can trace the origins of risk-based thinking back through time in many different areas of human activity besides insurance and heavy engineering. Judith Green (1997), for example, gives an outstanding analysis of our interpretation of 'accidents' and their transformation from acts of fate to predictable and hence preventable occurrences.

Nonetheless, as the UK Cabinet Office's Strategy Unit has observed (Cabinet Office 2002), in the context of the last century:

explicit risk management is a relatively recent phenomenon outside certain specialised areas. It developed earlier in the financial sector (insurance, banking), the military, and in audit and health and safety functions. But it is now developing steadily as a mainstream management activity across both public and private sectors. Risk has moved from being seen as a technical subject to being viewed as central to managing the whole organisation.

Why the present-day interest in risk-based decision making?

This is a complex question. However, it is worthwhile to consider some of the motivations. The basic issue is that human beings and human society are at all times faced by a multitude of risks. Some of these are accepted because of the benefits associated with them, for example, we sometimes use 'risky' transport systems to get from one place to another. Ideally, perhaps, we would wish to reduce all of the risks that we face, but this is not possible for two reasons. One is resources – we have not, either individually or as a society, the time or money to tackle all risks. Second, reducing risks sometimes means that we lose some benefit of an activity. Thus, if transport systems were designed never to exceed, say, 30 km per hour we would all be safer but it would take longer to complete journeys, so time, a valued commodity, would be lost.

 Activity 2.3

Write down an example of where you personally make a compromise between exposing yourself to some risk and receiving a benefit. How do you justify this compromise? Do the same for a risk that is the responsibility of an organization such as your employer or your municipality.

 Feedback

There are countless examples to choose from. Many sports that people play present high injury risks which would not normally be tolerated, but people still play them because they get enjoyment out of it and because it keeps them fit. Many people smoke cigarettes while fully aware of the health risks, but apparently accept these in exchange for the sensation it provides. Organizations also take risks when they invest effort and resources in projects, since future success can never be guaranteed. In fact, you could say that every action, not excluding the implementation of a new environmental health policy, introduces risk, but without taking such chances, there would be no opportunity for progress.

Thoughts such as these lead us inevitably to the issue of prioritization which is of fundamental importance to policy makers. This, in turn, brings up the matter of how to prioritize. It could be argued, and often is, that if we are unable to reduce all risks, perhaps we should seek to control those risks which are greatest and likely to cause the most harm. This approach to prioritization, however, is open to question. For example, some risks require a large investment of resources to bring about a meaningful reduction, whereas others may be reduced with fairly meagre investment (of time, materials, effort and money). Therefore, a preferred system of prioritization might be to measure the ratio of the benefits of a risk-reducing measure (note: risk-reducing measures are sometimes called 'interventions') to its cost in terms of time, effort and money.

It is a fact that governments, companies, institutions, municipalities and ultimately individuals are all interested in the efficient use of tax revenue resources, and this applies even in the context of health. What this implies is that there is a *prima facie* interest in investing in health measures that produce the largest benefit per unit of resource consumed. Interestingly, research by Tammy Tengs in the USA (Tengs et al. 1995) has investigated the cost and the effectiveness in prolonging life of 500 life-saving interventions.

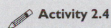 **Activity 2.4**

Table 2.1 shows a sample of the results from the work of Tengs and colleagues. What inferences can you draw from this?

Table 2.1 The estimated cost of a life-year saved by various interventions

Intervention	Cost ($)
Influenza vaccination	500
Pneumonia vaccination for people 65+	2200
Chlorination of drinking water	3100
All medical interventions	19 000
All aviation sector interventions	23 000
AZT for people with AIDS	26 000
All consumer product safety interventions	68 000
All occupational safety and health interventions	88 000
Widen lanes on rural roads	150 000
Pneumonia vaccination for children age 2–4	160 000
Asbestos control in cement industry	1 900 000
All toxic chemical controls	2 800 000
All environmental interventions	7 600 000

continued

Table 2.1 *continued*

Intervention	Cost ($)
Strengthen buildings in earthquake-prone areas	18 000 000
Sickle cell screening for newborns	65 000 000
Radionuclide emission control at uranium fuel cycle facilities	34 000 000 000

Source: Tengs et al. (1995)

Note: Some of the entries are averages for sectors and some apply to specific interventions.

 Feedback

Table 2.1 shows the net resource cost per year of life saved by the named intervention. For example, the figure of $500 against influenza vaccination means that for every $500 spent on that measure, one extra year of life is gained by all those who received the treatment (it does not mean that each vaccination cost $500). The implications of the data in Table 2.1 are that there are very large differences in the cost-effectiveness of interventions, and therefore that more lives could be saved if resources were shifted away from those with a high cost per life-year figure.

This need to use the resources that we have efficiently and to maximum public benefit can be recognized throughout society. It is frequently, though with some notable exceptions, encountered in legislation, even legislation aimed at protecting health and the environment, as there is usually some sort of requirement to allocate resources efficiently. In Activity 1.3 you came across the word 'appropriate' in the context of environmental health policy principles. Here we are touching on one aspect of the word 'appropriate' – it refers to interventions which *inter alia* are cost-effective. Where there is not a requirement to allocate resources efficiently, space is usually provided for policy makers to introduce such considerations. The World Health Organization (WHO), for example, when it recommended air quality guidelines as a basis for protecting human health from adverse effects of air pollution, stated that their purpose was to provide guidance to governments in making risk management decisions. The WHO went on to emphasize that the guidelines should not be regarded as mandatory, but should be considered in the context of prevailing exposure levels, and social, economic and cultural conditions (WHO 1987). In other words, the priority to be given to the achievement of the guidelines was seen as being subject to other local needs, which might be more important, including efficiency.

The need to use risk-based approaches in public policy decision making can be observed implicitly or explicitly in a wide variety of legislation, and in the procedures of international agencies, such as the International Atomic Energy Agency (IAEA) and conventions such as SOLAS (Safety of Life at Sea).

Risk-based requirements are now mandatory in many countries. In the UK, the statute governing health and safety in the workplace (the 1974 Health and Safety at Work Act) adopts a risk-based approach, as does the more recent Management of Health and Safety at Work Regulations 1999. Likewise, in Europe, the Workplace

Safety Directive, introduced in 1993, has regulations covering health and safety management which specifically require a risk-based approach. Requirements of this kind can be found in many countries.

The health sector itself is also a prime candidate for such methodologies. As Arnold Relman, former editor of the *New England Journal of Medicine*, argued in 1988, in order to properly organize health care in the future, it will be necessary

to know much more about the relative costs, safety, and effectiveness of all the things physicians do or employ in the diagnosis, treatment, and prevention of disease. Armed with these facts, physicians will be in a much stronger position to advise their patients and determine the use of medical resources, payers will be better able to decide what to pay for, and the public will have a better understanding of what is available and what they want.

 Activity 2.5

Can you think of any statutes, requirements or advice applying in your region that incorporate the need for a risk-based approach? What are they?

 Feedback

The requirement for a risk-based approach may not be explicit. Nonetheless, if you look at legislation, codes of practice or advice in any of the fields of occupational health and safety, consumer protection, food safety, transport safety or environmental health, you might well find the use of words that imply that while controls are expected, they are only required if it is 'reasonable', 'practicable', 'cost-effective', etc. to apply them. Implicit in the use of such words is that someone has assessed the risk reduction benefit of an intervention and compared it with the cost to see if it is reasonable. Sometimes there are absolute requirements which say that an intervention must be made irrespective of cost, but this is unusual.

Important changes from past to present

Given the history outlined above, and the rapidly changing times in which we live, it should not be surprising that contemporary ways of thinking about and coping with risks are different from earlier times. In the last century alone, major changes have occurred in the nature and perception of risks. The following edited extract from Vince Covello and Jeryl Mumpower (1985) lists nine changes which they observed. Though based on US experience, you may find some parallels with your own country. You may well find some differences too, which should also be of interest.

 Activity 2.6

As you read the following edited version of the changes in thinking about risk identified by Covello and Mumpower (1985), make notes on whether the changes identified are also apparent, or not, within your own country. If some factors do not apply, suggest reasons why that might be so.

- prioritizing the allocation of resources available for environmental improvement;
- investigating the environmental health risks associated with new developments in the built environment;
- investigating health risks (and benefits) of policy changes;
- assessing the impact on health of legislative change;
- making recommendations in situations where there are no relevant environmental standards or guidelines;
- investigating situations where there is a high level of public concern.

Summary

Risk assessment is now seen as an important tool for bringing about effective and efficient environmental health policies. In this chapter you looked at the history of risk assessment and noted a number of factors which slowed its initial development, and also at influences which are bringing about present-day change in the way society deals with risk. The strength of these influences, and hence the need to accommodate them, will vary from place to place and this should be kept in mind when thinking about policy development.

References

Cabinet Office (2002) Risk: improving government's capability to handle risk and uncertainty. http://www.strategy.gov.uk/work_areas/risk/index.asp

Commonwealth of Australia (2002) *Environmental Health Risk Assessment: Guidelines for Assessing Human Health Risks from Environmental Hazards*. Canberra: HMSO.

Covello VT and Mumpower J (1985) Risk analysis and risk management: an historical perspective. *Risk Analysis* 5(2): 103–20.

David FN (1962) *Games, Gods and Gambling*. London: Griffin & Co.

Green J (1997) *Risk and Misfortune: The Social Construction of Accidents*. London: UCL Press.

Grier B (1980) *One Thousand Years of Mathematical Psychology*. Madison, WI: Society for Mathematical Psychology.

Paustenbach DJ (1989) *The Risk Assessment of Environmental and Human Health Hazards*. New York: John Wiley and Sons, Ltd.

Relman AS (1988) Assessment and accountability: the third revolution in medical care. *New England Journal of Medicine* 319: 1220–2.

Tengs T et al. (1995) Five hundred life saving interventions and their cost effectiveness, *Risk Analysis* 15(3): 369–90.

World Health Organization (1987) *Air Quality Guidelines for Europe*. Copenhagen: WHO European Office.

SECTION 2

Assessing environmental health risks

3 | A model for human health risk assessment

Overview

In the previous chapter you saw how risk assessment had moved centre stage by the twenty-first century as a tool for the management of environmental health risks and the formulation of health policy. This chapter will introduce the classic quantitative risk assessment model in the field of environmental health, and give an outline description of each component.

Learning objectives

By the end of this chapter, you will be better able to:

- **describe the classic four-stage risk assessment model**
- **distinguish between risk assessment and risk management**
- **define key terms.**

Key terms

Dose A stated quantity or concentration of a substance to which an organism is exposed over either a continuous or an intermittent period. Dose is most commonly measured in units of milligrams per kilogram of body weight of the receiver (mg/kg bw).

Dose–response assessment The determination of the relationship between administered doses and the incidence or severity of the associated adverse effects.

Environmental agent Any chemical, biological or physical substance, or social factor, which is under investigation.

Exposure assessment A qualitative or quantitative estimation of the magnitude, frequency and duration of exposure of the general population, subgroups or individuals, to hazardous substances or situations.

Exposure pathway The means by which risk agents come into contact with target organisms, e.g. via drinking water, inhalation, dermal contact, or physical proximity, etc.

Hazard A factor or exposure that may adversely affect health.

Hazard identification The identification of adverse health or environmental effects which could be associated with an agent or situation should exposure arise.

Risk The probability that an event will occur within a specified time.

Risk assessment The activity of estimating the potential impact of a chemical, biological, physical or other hazard upon a target individual, group or population.

Risk characterization A synthesis and summary of information about a potentially hazardous situation that addresses the needs and interests of decision makers and of interested and affected parties. Risk characterization is a prelude to decision making and depends on an iterative, analytic deliberative process.

Risk management The use of risk assessment in combination with socio-economic and political inputs to evaluate and select measures to manage risk.

The nature of human health risk assessment

In 1983, the US National Research Council (NRC 1983) published an early and influential book (referred to as 'the Red Book') on the nature of risk assessment as applied to public health. It opened by making an important distinction between *risk assessment* and *risk management*. Risk assessment was seen as referring to the use of factual information to define the health effects resulting from the exposure of individual persons or populations to hazardous agents or situations. Risk management was seen as the process of weighing policy alternatives and selecting the most appropriate action. That is, risk management required the integration of risk assessment data with social, economic, and political concerns prior to any decision being made. You will notice some similarity to the World Health Organization's position on air quality guidelines as described in Chapter 2. The WHO also saw the need for risk management decisions to reflect local priorities in the form of economic, social and political circumstances.

There is good reason for this. Suppose, for example, a quantitative risk assessment of discharges from a factory indicated that they might result in some health detriment to the local population. While in the ideal world this hazard would surely be eliminated, the reality might be that the factory provides employment for the community, and to control its emissions would undermine its viability. Thus there is a trade-off to be made between environmental health and other outcomes related to economic welfare, which in turn have implications for employment, housing, diet and health itself. Thus, risk management decisions often have to take account of other issues, some of which may fall outside the technical arena.

You may conclude that risk assessment alone, while it can well be a prerequisite for policy formulation, is not sufficient on its own. In recent times this separation of risk assessment and risk management, as you will see in Chapter 17, has been somewhat eroded, but for the time being we will use it as a working model. This separation is shown in Figure 3.1.

✎ Activity 3.1

What do you think are the advantages of separating risk assessment from risk management?

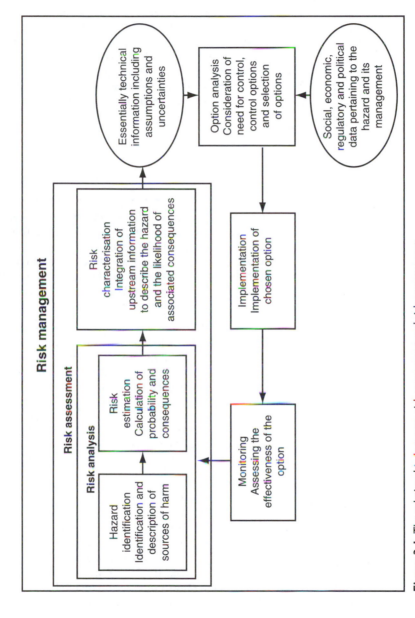

Figure 3.1 The relationship between risk assessment and risk management

Source: Ball (2000)

↻ **Feedback**

The risk assessment stage is primarily about technical information and analysis and is the area of people skilled in those matters, for example, epidemiologists, toxicologists, physicians and risk analysts. The information used is usually perceived as quantitative and objective. In contrast, policy formulation and decision making require many other inputs, some of which are far more qualitative and subjective. By separating the two functions, the technical experts are able to fulfil their role, which is often difficult enough, without the added complexity of the value judgements that are present in decision making. Furthermore, potentially important socio-economic issues do not get subsumed into the technical process where, conceivably, they might be lost.

Note that according to this model, human health risk assessment is a predominantly technical matter. You will return to this later.

The nature of risk

The term 'risk' has been used by numerous different professions as well as by the public and has come to mean many different things (Althaus 2005). Although attempts have been made to encourage standardized definitions, it is unlikely that a common usage will be achieved within the near future. Consequently, users of this term will need to be clear in their own minds and to make clear to others the particular definition they are using. You will also find that the meaning which you yourself attach to this term will change depending upon the circumstances.

According to common usage, 'risk' is more or less synonymous with 'danger', though danger itself is an ill-defined term, like 'safety', and best avoided if possible. In environmental health protection, the definition of risk most often used follows from that used in engineering and allied fields, where it refers to the probability of some specified form of harm being realized. For example, the probability of an earthquake of specified magnitude occurring at a particular location during, say, the next year, or of a chemical release of a certain size from a manufacturing plant during a specified time period. It could also refer to the probability that cancer will occur in a given population in a specified time interval following exposure to a chemical.

Probability itself is a mathematical expression of the likelihood of a chance event and can be expressed in a number of different ways, for example, as an annual or lifetime risk of dying, of contracting some disease, or of suffering an injury as a result, say, of an accident. It could also refer to the risk of a one-off event, for example, a tsunami. Table 3.1 lists some health risks, expressed as annual risks, which pertained a few years ago in the United Kingdom (BMA 1987). Alternatively, as an example of a *lifetime* risk, the WHO says that the lifetime risk of cancer from exposure to hexavalent chromium is estimated to be 4×10^{-2} (i.e. 4 per cent) for continuous exposure to an air concentration of 1 µg per m^3 (WHO 1987).

Table 3.1 The risks of an individual dying from specified causes in any one year, UK data 1980s

Cause	Risk
Smoking 10 cigarettes a day	one in 200
All natural causes, age 40	one in 850
Any kind of violence or poisoning	one in 3300
Influenza	one in 5000
Accident on the road	one in 8000
Leukaemia	one in 12 500
Playing soccer	one in 25 000
Accident at home	one in 26 000
Accident at work	one in 43 500
Working with radiation in nuclear industry	one in 57 000
Homicide	one in 100 000
Accident on railway	one in 500 000
Hit by lightning	one in 10 000 000
Release of radiation from nuclear facility	one in 10 000 000

Source: British Medical Association (1987)

Other terms that you will encounter include hazard. Hazard is usually defined as the property of a substance, or a situation, that could lead to harm. Arsenic in drinking water could constitute a hazard, as could an unprotected well shaft.

It is worthwhile being aware that the term risk could have strikingly different meanings for other users. In the world of banking, for example, 'risk' is differentiated from 'uncertainty' and is sometimes used to indicate that it is possible to make a precise estimate of the probability of an outcome. In the field of economic appraisal, 'risk' could mean the possibility of more than one outcome occurring (RCEP 1998).

Individual and population risk

It is necessary to be familiar with other uses of the word 'risk'. Here we will consider 'individual risk' and 'population risk', though other kinds will be examined later. Individual risks, as the name implies, are those risks which apply to an hypothetical individual with either the characteristics of a typical person, or of a highly exposed or particularly susceptible person, depending on the purpose. Individual risk is most often described in terms of the risk per year or per lifetime of some specified event, such as contracting a particular disease.

Population risk usually relates to the number of adverse health effects (e.g. fatalities, cancers, injuries, etc.) expected in a population over a specified time period, or the rate of adverse effects for a given location or group of people (Covello and Merkhofer 1993).

Steps in environmental health risk assessment

As described in the Red Book, and adopted in similar form by other agencies worldwide, health risk assessment can be divided into four major stages (Figure 3.2):

- hazard identification
- dose–response assessment
- exposure assessment
- risk characterization.

It is appropriate to consider these stages in some detail.

Hazard identification

Hazard identification refers to the process of determining whether a particular chemical or physical agent has the capacity to cause an increase in the incidence of a health condition (cancer, respiratory disease, injury, etc.). It is usually applied to human receptors, but, as with the other stages of risk assessment, could be applied to non-humans. It involves characterizing the nature and strength of the evidence of causation. This is because there is often no straight answer to the question of whether an agent is harmful. In fact, the question is often restated in terms of the effects on laboratory animals or other test systems, but this requires extrapolation from one species to another and probably from one dose to another, and so although it does present evidence, it is inconclusive.

Dose–response assessment

This is the process of characterizing the relationship between the dose of an agent administered or received and the incidence of an adverse health effect in exposed populations. The process considers important factors such as intensity of exposure, the age distribution of those exposed, and possibly other variables that might affect response, such as gender and lifestyle. Dose–response relationships mainly are based on toxicological studies involving animal testing and so extrapolation from high to low doses is often required as well as between species, say, from animals to humans.

Exposure assessment

Exposure assessment is the process of measuring or estimating the intensity, frequency and duration of exposure to an agent present in the environment. In its complete form it should describe the magnitude, duration and route of exposure and the characteristics of those exposed. Exposure assessment is often the poor relation of the risk assessment process, as it is often neglected, but it is important because it can often be used at the risk management stage to predict the effects of alternative control options.

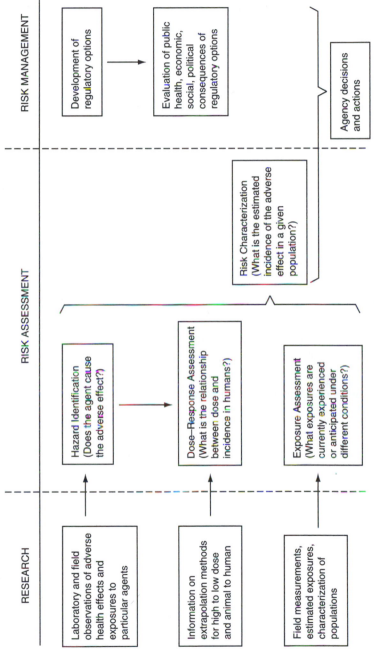

Figure 3.2 The classical risk assessment process illustrating the four stages of risk assessment and their relationship to information inputs and contribution to policy formulation
Source: NRC (1983)

Risk characterization

This is traditionally described as the process of estimating the incidence of a specified health effect under the various conditions of human or animal exposure described in the exposure assessment. It is carried out by combining exposure and dose–response information. Uncertainties should be specified.

Summary

Environmental health risks are conventionally assessed using a four-stage model involving hazard identification, dose–response assessment, exposure assessment and risk characterization. This information is used to inform risk management decisions and public health policy, but does not bring it about on its own. A number of definitional problems exist within the field and you should always be careful when defining what terms mean in specific circumstances and what others mean by them.

References

Althaus CE (2005) A disciplinary perspective on the epistemological status of risk. *Risk Analysis* 25(3): 567–88.

Ball DJ (2000) Risks of injury: an overview, in Harries M, McLatchie G, Williams C and King J (eds) *ABC of Sports Medicine*. London: BMJ Books.

British Medical Association (1987) *Living with Risk*. Chichester: John Wiley & Sons Ltd.

Covello VT and Merkhofer MW (1993) *Risk Assessment Methods: Approaches for Assessing Health and Environmental Risks*. New York: Plenum Press.

NRC (1983) *Risk Assessment in the Federal Government: Managing the Process*. Washington, DC: National Academy Press.

Royal Commission on Environmental Pollution (1998) *Setting Environmental Standards*. London: The Stationery Office.

World Health Organization (1987) *Air Quality Guidelines for Europe*. Copenhagen: WHO.

4 Hazard identification

Overview

In Chapter 3 you saw how the four-stage model of human health risk assessment is constructed. This chapter will describe in greater detail the first stage of that process – hazard identification. You will be introduced to some relevant terminology, and proceed to consider the two most important techniques of hazard identification for environmental health purposes. These are toxicological studies and epidemiology. The approaches are very different, but they complement each other remarkably well.

Learning objectives

By the end of this chapter, you will be better able to:

- **describe the process of hazard identification**
- **compare and contrast the main techniques for identifying environmental hazards**
- **understand the meaning of commonly used terms.**

Key terms

Acute exposure A short exposure, typically of hours or minutes, possibly at a high level.

Carcinogen Any chemical or physical agent able to induce cancer in living organisms.

Case-control study An observational study starting with the identification of a group of cases and controls. The level of exposure to the risk factor of interest can then be measured (retrospectively) and compared.

Chronic exposure An exposure of long duration, months or years, and usually to a low concentration.

Cohort A group or population that share a common characteristic.

Cohort study A follow-up observational study where groups of individuals are defined on the basis of their exposure to a certain suspected risk factor for a disease.

Confounding variable (confounder) A variable that is associated with the exposure under study and is also a risk factor for the outcome in its own right.

Cross-sectional study A study design where exposure and outcome are measured at the same time.

Ecological fallacy The effects measured in groups may not be applicable at the level of individuals.

Epidemiology The study of the distribution and determinants of health states or events in specified populations, and the application of this study to the control of health problems.

Incidence The frequency of new cases in a defined population during a specified period of time.

in vitro A laboratory test using living cells taken from an organism.

in vivo A laboratory test carried out on living organisms such as whole animals or human volunteers.

LD_{50} The dose that when administered to animals in a test is lethal to 50 per cent.

Mutagen An agent that can cause genetic damage to individual cells.

Prevalence The frequency of existing cases in a defined population at a particular point in time (point prevalence), or over a given period of time (period prevalence), as a proportion of the total population.

Teratogen An agent which can induce congenital anomalies in a developing foetus.

Toxicology The study of the adverse effects of chemicals on living organisms.

Poisons and other hazardous compounds

The first stage in the classic model of risk assessment is the identification of hazards. As in Table 1.1, hazards come in many forms but this model is primarily concerned with human health hazards arising from exposure to chemical or other agents. You will be familiar with terms like 'hazard' and 'poison' but may not be aware of their particular meanings in specialist circles.

 Activity 4.1

As you read the following edited passage by Alice Ottoboni (1991), former toxicologist for the California State Department of Public Health, note how key terms such as 'poison' and 'hazard' are defined. You will also encounter the technical term, LD_{50}, widely used in the study of toxicology.

When you have read the article, you should have an understanding of the meaning of these terms. You should also be able to reflect upon the following quote attributed to the famous sixteenth-century Swiss physician, Paracelsus: 'What is it that is not a poison? All things are poison and nothing is without poison. It is the dose only that makes a thing not a poison.' Is Paracelsus' quote consistent with modern terminology?

 Definitions of poison, hazard and toxicity

A chemical that causes illness or death is often referred to as a poison. This concept is erroneous and has resulted in a great deal of confusion in the public mind about the nature of the toxic action of chemicals. Poisons are chemicals that produce illness or death when taken in very small quantities. Legally, a poison is defined as a chemical that has an LD_{50} of 50 milligrams, or less, per kilogram of body weight. An LD_{50} is the quantity of chemical administered in one dose that is lethal for 50 percent of test animals within a 14-day period. LD means lethal dose and the subscript 50 refers to the percentage of the animals for which the dose was lethal.

Fifty mg/kg is equal to approximately three-fourths of a teaspoon for an average adult and about one-eighth of a teaspoon for an average 2-year-old child. There are very few chemicals that are lethal in such small quantities. Thus, there are not many chemicals that can be classed as poisons, yet there are many, many chemicals that are capable of causing illness or death. Even among the dreaded pesticides, the majority do not fall within the category of poison. Therefore, to consider only poisons are harmful or that harmful chemicals are, of necessity, poisons is a misleading and dangerous assumption.

LD_{50}s are almost always related to the toxicity of chemicals; however, chemicals that are corrosive can also kill, especially when they are ingested. Thus, a corrosive chemical, like a toxic one, will be classed as a poison if it is lethal in doses of 50 mg/kg or less. A good example of chemicals that are labelled as poisons because of their corrosiveness are the well-known drain-opener products that are found in many kitchens. One might consider it splitting hairs to distinguish between corrosiveness and toxicity as a cause of death. Although the distinction has little significance in human terms, it is one that must be made in a proper study of the harmful effects of chemicals.

Another distinction that should be made is the difference between toxicity and hazard. The latter has come into common use as a synonym for the former. Actually hazard is a much more complex concept than toxicity because it includes conditions of use. The hazard presented by a chemical has two components: (1) the inherent ability of a chemical to do harm by virtue of its explosiveness, flammability, corrosiveness, toxicity, and so forth; and (2) the ease with which contact can be established between the chemical and the object of concern . . . For example, an extremely toxic chemical, such as strychnine, when sealed in an unopenable vial, can be handled freely by people with no chance that a poisoning will occur. Its toxicity has not changed, but it presents no hazard because no contact can be established between the chemical and people. Conversely, a chemical that is not highly toxic can be very hazardous when used in a manner that makes it available for accidental ingestion.

 Feedback

> Paracelsus was clearly using a different definition of 'poison' from that now favoured. Nonetheless, he was a man far ahead of his time. His point here, which is valid, is that the effects of an agent are dependent upon the dose received, something which you will explore further in Chapter 5. The passage by Alice Ottoboni shows that commonly used terms, like 'poison' and 'hazard', have special significance for professionals.

Methods of hazard identification

Hazard identification, at least in the area of environmental health, uses three basic approaches. These are:

1   *in vivo* animal testing based upon toxicological methods;
2   epidemiological studies of human groups;
3   other tests.

The first two are currently the most widely used and are now described further. 'Other tests' include, for example, *in vitro* tests on isolated cell systems, or studies involving the comparison of the molecular structures of suspect compounds with those of known toxins.

Toxicological studies

Toxicology is the science that investigates the adverse systemic effects of chemicals, that is, the effects upon the whole body. Hazard identification by toxicity testing is mainly reliant upon *in vivo* testing on animals conducted according to standard protocols. A range of tests are used, the main ones being (Commonwealth of Australia 2002):

- *acute toxicity tests*. These investigate the effects of single doses of a substance and commonly are used to identify the medium lethal dose, or LD_{50} over a 14-day post-dosing period.
- *sub-chronic toxicity tests*. These investigate the effects in the short term of repeated doses.
- *chronic toxicity tests*. These are studies of the effects of long-term exposure to an agent.
- *reproductive toxicity tests*. These are designed to identify the effects of test substances on the reproductive performance of males and females.
- *mutagenicity tests*. These are designed to determine if test chemicals can cause gene or chromosomal mutations that can be passed to another generation.
- *carcinogenicity tests*. These seek to determine the cancer-causing potential of an agent.

Ethical considerations rule out the deliberate exposure of people to hazardous agents except in the case of clinical trials with volunteers. As a result, toxicity data for humans are often unavailable, other than in the aftermath of accidents such as those at Bhopal, Seveso, and Minamata.

 Activity 4.2

Toxicological testing is performed on animals (itself now raising ethical questions in some countries). However, this has its own drawbacks. Note some of the factors that you think might limit its usefulness.

 Feedback

The main problem is uncertainties in extrapolating from animals to humans, and in extrapolating from the typically high doses given to animals over short periods of time in laboratory tests, and the generally much lower doses experienced by humans over long periods in the environment. Exposure pathways may also differ.

Human equivalent doses have traditionally been derived from animal data by the relatively crude method of scaling the dose in proportion to body weight, although in some cases more sophisticated methods are available to provide biologically equivalent doses, though these methods are also prone to a range of uncertainties.

Even in situations where human data are available, as, for example, in the unintended exposure of workers to toxic materials, extrapolation to the general public may be problematic. This is because occupational data often apply to a relatively healthy, mainly male workforce within a specific age-band, whereas the general public are not restricted in this way.

Epidemiological studies

Epidemiological studies provide a very important complement to toxicology in the identification of chemical and other hazards, and in the case of microbiological hazards, epidemiology is the principal method. Epidemiology is concerned with the study of the distribution and causes of health states in specified populations, with its ultimate purpose being to help in the identification of health-related interventions. It is very dependent upon the appropriate and exacting use of statistical methods.

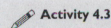 **Activity 4.3**

The following abridged passage (Commonwealth of Australia 2002) provides a brief but valuable review of the four main categories of epidemiological study. It is important to understand the strengths and limitations of the different methods and of epidemiology in general. In particular, the ability to make links between cause and effect. As you read it, make a note of the relative contributions to hazard identification made by epidemiology and toxicology.

 Types of environmental epidemiological study

In practical terms there are four main categories of study:

* case-control studies
* cross-sectional studies
* cohort (longitudinal) studies, and
* ecological studies (including a sub-group known as time-series studies).

In case-control studies, exposure and other attributes of cases of the disease under investigation are compared with those from a suitable control or comparison group of persons unaffected by the condition, and analysed to yield effect estimates.

Cross-sectional studies measure the prevalence of disease and measure exposure and effect at the same time.

Cohort studies follow cohorts or groups of individuals, defined in terms of their exposures, over time to see if there are differences in the development of new cases of the disease of interest (or other health outcome) between the groups with and without exposure. Such studies can be carried out by either reviewing past studies (retrospective) or by tracking people into the future (prospective cohort). The essential feature of these longitudinal studies is that for each individual prior exposure information can be related to subsequent disease experience.

Ecological studies involve the investigation of a group of people such as those living within a geographical area such as a region or state. For example, place and time of residence may be used to create surrogate measures of the real exposure of interest. Rates of disease and average exposure levels to a particular agent are determined independently, and on a group basis. This may give rise to a spurious apparent correlation, called the ecological fallacy. Because it is not ascertained whether individuals who have been exposed to the agent are the same individuals who developed the disease, statements about causal relationships are inappropriate. However, ecological studies are relatively inexpensive for linking available health data sets and environmental information and are useful for hypothesis generation. Examples of ecological studies are the assessments of the relationship between tobacco sales in different countries and lung cancer rates, and fluoride in water and dental caries.

A subset of ecological studies, known as time-series studies, is regarded as very helpful in understanding the influence of short-term fluctuations in, say, air pollutants on day-to-day changes in population morbidity and mortality after controlling for factors such as season and air temperature. However, disentangling the effects of individual pollutants as measured in a mixture such as urban air pollution can be difficult . . .

Epidemiological studies are rarely definitive and a single study cannot establish causality. A 'weight of evidence' approach is generally required, involving the interpretation of all available information.

Overall, epidemiological studies, depending upon their design, may serve two purposes: hypothesis-generation or assessment of a causal relationship. Their ability to evaluate a causal relationship may be limited by a lack of control of potential confounders (confounders are factors which distort the effect of the agent of interest) or a lack of statistical power (usually because of limited sample sizes).

 Feedback

A clear advantage of epidemiological studies is that there is no need to extrapolate between species. This would be particularly problematic if the interest were in, say, mental functioning, or behavioural or subjective effects, but is always an issue. On the other hand, epidemiological studies are more vulnerable to uncertainties in both exposure and dose, which can be tightly controlled in toxicological work. Toxicology is also necessary for confirming causal mechanisms. And when it comes to dose–response relationships, the subject of the next chapter, epidemiological studies can be seen to measure exposure–response rather than dose–response.

Summary

In the field of environmental health there are two principal methods of hazard identification: toxicology and epidemiology. Toxicology is mainly reliant upon animal testing, whereas epidemiology acquires knowledge by the study of the occurrence of symptoms and disease in human populations. In this chapter you have learned about the basics of the approaches and some of their strengths and limitations. In moving on to policy formulation, it is important to have an awareness of the strengths and limitations of the various information inputs.

References

Commonwealth of Australia (2002) *Environmental Health Risk Assessment: Guidelines for Assessing Human Health Risks from Environmental Hazards*. Canberra: Commonwealth of Australia.

Covello VT and Merkhofer MW (1993) *Risk Assessment Methods: Approaches for Assessing Health and Environmental Risks*. New York: Plenum Press.

National Research Council (1983) *Risk Assessment in the Federal Government: Managing the Process*. Washington, DC: National Academy Press.

Ottoboni MA (1991) *The Dose Makes the Poison*. New York: Van Nostrand Reinhold.

Paustenbach DJ (1989) *The Risk Assessment of Environmental Hazards*. New York: John Wiley & Sons Ltd.

The dose–response relationship

Overview

In Chapter 4 you saw how chemical hazards are identified. This chapter introduces you to the next stage of the classical environmental health risk assessment model, namely, the determination of the dose–response relationship. As before, there is a fair amount of terminology involved but this is inevitable in dealing with a multi-disciplinary subject such as environmental health policy. Here you will be examining how toxic agents are assessed, and in particular, the different approaches used in assessing agents that pose a finite risk at any level of exposure, however small, and those which are harmful only above a certain dose. As you will find out, this distinction is of fundamental importance for the development of risk management as applied to health policy.

Learning objectives

By the end of this chapter, you will be better able to:

- **describe how scientists go about defining dose–response curves for toxic agents**
- **identify the different approaches to defining 'safe' levels of exposure for threshold and non-threshold agents**
- **discuss the strengths and limitations of the approaches and the results derived.**

Key terms

Acceptable daily intake (ADI) The daily intake of a chemical which, during a lifetime, appears to be without appreciable risk. Usually measured in mg/kg/day.

Carcinogenesis The process of the origination, causation and development of malignant tumours.

Deoxyribonucleic acid (DNA) The molecule in which the genetic blueprint for living cells is encoded.

Genotoxic A chemical that can cause damage in genetic material leading to heritable changes.

Linear no threshold hypothesis The presumption that risk is linearly related to dose at low doses for non-threshold agents.

Lowest observed adverse effect level The lowest experimental or observed concentration or amount of a substance that causes adverse alterations in target organisms.

Multi-hit model Dose–response models that assume that more than one interaction with a toxic material at the molecular level is necessary to cause an effect.

No observed adverse effect level (NOAEL) The highest dose at which no significant adverse effects are noticed in a population.

One-hit model Dose–response models that assume that a response occurs after a target has been impacted once at the molecular level by a biologically effective dose.

Reference dose An estimate of the highest daily dosage of a risk agent that is unlikely to produce an appreciable harmful effect in humans.

Safety factor A single factor or several factors used to derive an acceptable intake of a chemical.

Stochastic A random statistical phenomenon.

Threshold The lowest dose or exposure level which will produce a toxic effect.

Assessing the health consequences of exposures

As discussed in Chapter 3, hazards can be identified via the disciplines of toxicology and epidemiology. As you are now aware, that marked the first stage of the classical health risk assessment model for environmental health. The aim is now to introduce the primary method of relating exposures to some specified agent to an adverse health effect. This is achieved by use of a dose–response relationship, which simply relates dose, as a measure of exposure, to an adverse health response.

Figure 5.1 shows a hypothetical dose–response curve as might have been derived from toxicological studies. In this graph, the ordinate (y-axis) records the percentage of the exposed population exhibiting an adverse consequence. Three curves are shown to clarify that individual toxins may have multiple adverse effects. Note that typically the curves have an 'S-shape'.

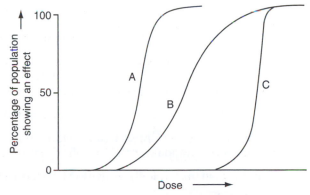

Figure 5.1 Hypothetical dose–response curves for a single chemical agent. If an agent causes more than one effect (three in this example) there will be multiple curves.

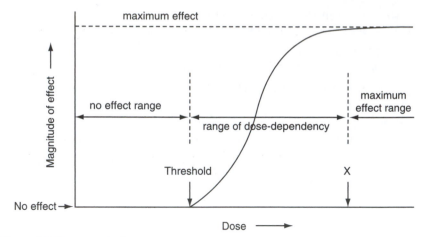

Figure 5.2 Features of a dose–response curve

Figure 5.2 looks at an individual dose–response curve in more detail. Note that here the ordinate measures the magnitude of a specified effect in a typical individual. For all doses above a certain dose (denoted X in Figure 5.2), the maximum effect is exhibited. Below this there is a range where the magnitude of the effect depends upon the dose received. Importantly, there is also a threshold below which there is no effect. Thresholds are believed to exist for some agents because of the ability of the body to metabolize or excrete a toxin, or to repair damage, up to a certain dose.

Thresholds and safety factors

The threshold approach has been used for over half a century to identify doses at which humans would not be expected to exhibit adverse effects. Traditional toxicological procedures define a safe level of exposure for humans as *some fraction* of the maximum dose level at which there is no observed effect. There are two terms that you need to be familiar with. The lowest dose which leads to an observable effect is known as the 'lowest observed effect level' (LOEL). The maximum dose without effect is referred to as the 'no observed adverse effect level' (NOAEL). Note the inclusion of the word 'adverse'. This is because some exposures create observable effects but these are not thought to be harmful, for example, one glass of beer.

The question now arises as to the fraction by which the NOAEL should be multiplied in order to define the level of dose which is 'safe'. Bearing in mind that most dose–response curves are based upon animal tests, it is customary to use a fraction of $\frac{1}{10}$ to allow for the fact that humans might be ten times more sensitive than the test animals. This *interspecies* factor is clearly somewhat arbitrary – it is a rule of thumb. Normally, however, the fraction applied (often known as the 'safety factor') is smaller than this; typically $\frac{1}{100}$ is used, i.e. a further factor of $\frac{1}{10}$ is introduced. This is to allow for further uncertainty associated with the variable sensitivity within the human population, that is, *intraspecies* variability, to specific agents. For example, children or people with pre-existing health problems may be more vulnerable than the average member of the population to a certain hazardous agent. Further allowances might also be made depending on the severity of the consequence of exposure, and the quantity and quality of the available scientific data on which the assessment is based. So if an agent has particularly insidious or uncertain consequences, a further judgemental factor might be incorporated.

 Activity 5.1

One shortcoming of the threshold and safety factor approach is that the potentially useful information provided by the slope of the dose–response curve in the region of the threshold is not used. In what way could this information be useful?

 Feedback

A moderate safety factor may provide an adequate safety margin if the dose–response curve is steep in the region of the threshold dose, but not if the gradient is shallow. The choice of safety factor could have economic implications, so it is important to try and gauge it appropriately.

Having decided upon the safety factor, say $\frac{1}{100}$, the NOAEL is then multiplied by this factor to yield various other related parameters which are used in specifying 'safe' levels:

- *Acceptable daily intake (ADI)*. The daily intake of a chemical which, during a lifetime, appears to be without appreciable risk. ADIs are usually expressed in mg/kg-body weight/day but may have different units depending on the exposure route.
- *Tolerable daily intake (TDI)*. An estimate of the daily intake of a substance which can occur over a lifetime without appreciable health risk. TDI is used in relation to contaminants which should not be present, whereas ADI is used in the context of contaminants that are present because they were deliberately used, such as pesticides on food crops.
- *Tolerable weekly intake (TWI)*.
- *Reference dose (RfD)*. An estimate of the daily exposure (mg/kg/day) to the general population that is likely to be without an appreciable risk of deleterious effects during a lifetime of exposure.

Non-threshold agents

Note that the use of a safety factor to determine acceptable human exposure levels relies upon the existence of a threshold dose below which adverse effects do not occur. However, the existence of a threshold below which there are no effects is not accepted for some compounds, notably, carcinogens. In the case of these materials, it is widely assumed that however small the dose, some risk of cancer remains.

Although biological arguments exist, for example, that DNA, while it may be susceptible to damage by a carcinogen, may have an effective self-repair mechanism at low doses, the threshold at which this eliminates risk is still likely to vary from one person to another, and its value is therefore very uncertain.

Another problem is that for agents that have either a very low or no threshold, there may be no animal test data available. Typically, dose–response curves are based on small numbers (for cost reasons) of test animals receiving high doses in short periods of time, but environmental health policy makers are mainly concerned with the quite different situation of large numbers of people being exposed to low doses over long periods.

✐ Activity 5.2

Figure 5.3 shows a situation which might be faced by an environmental health policy maker. The example is of exposure to ionizing radiation. Unusually, in this example, human dose–response data are available, based on studies of survivors of Hiroshima and Nagasaki, and from occupational exposures to high levels of radiation in uranium mines. This information provides the cluster of data in the top-right corner of Figure 5.3. However, these are clearly abnormal exposures, and if your task were to assess the risk of harm to a population exposed to much lower, background levels of radiation, as in the lower-left corner of Figure 5.3, how would you do this?

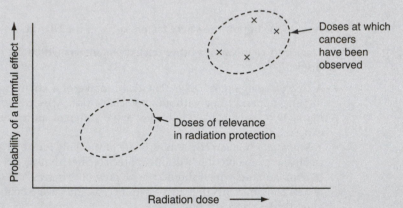

Figure 5.3 The problem of evidence that is not available. Health effect data may exist for high exposures but mainly the interest is in low exposures.

↻ Feedback

In dealing with ionizing radiation and some genotoxic carcinogens, it is assumed that there is no threshold. A non-threshold model has therefore to be adopted. Traditionally, non-threshold models assume a linear relationship between the lowest experimentally-observed dose and zero dose. This is known as the LNT (linear no threshold) hypothesis. Note, it is an hypothesis and is not scientifically proven, although there are scientific arguments that support this assumption. In general, scientists are discouraged from extrapolating outside of the range of measured data, though the environmental policy maker unfortunately has little choice in this matter.

Activity 5.3

What is the implication of the LNT hypothesis for the safety of humans exposed to ionizing radiation and chemical carcinogens, whether exposure occurs in the health service, industry, or from the natural background?

Feedback

The implication is far-reaching. It is that there is no such thing as a safe dose if 'safe' is taken as meaning zero risk. This means that policy makers have somehow to define levels of risk for non-threshold agents which are non-zero but somehow 'tolerable'. This is a major issue that you will encounter as you progress through this book.

Another important and debated issue involving the LNT hypothesis is the assumed linear relationship between dose and effect at doses outside the range for which data exist, either from animal tests or epidemiological studies. Figure 5.4 summarizes the situation. Data points are shown, but what does the curve really look like at low doses? Is it straight (b); supra-linear (a); sub-linear (c); or threshold (d)?

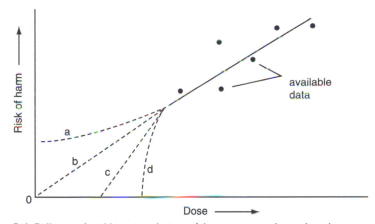

Figure 5.4 Different plausible extrapolations of dose–response data at low doses

Activity 5.4

The implications for policy makers of the above uncertainties of low-dose extrapolation models are discussed in the following abridged extracts which have been collated by Paustenbach (1989). As you read them, familiarize yourself with the dilemmas faced by scientists who are trying to provide useful information on which environmental policy makers may base their decisions.

Three views of implications for policy makers of uncertainties

Stochastic models are based on the premise that a positive response is the result of the random occurrence of one or more biological events. The one-hit model is based on the concept that a response will occur after the target site has been hit by a single biologically effective unit of dose. The multi-hit model is a direct extension of the one-hit model, assuming that more than one hit is required in order to induce a response. . . .

The shape of the dose–response curves for the above models in the low-dose region will have considerable impact on estimates of risk associated with low levels of exposure. For example, the one-hit model is linear at low doses and will thus generally provide relatively high estimates of risk at low dose levels. The multi-stage model is linear at low doses only in certain defined circumstances and is sub-linear otherwise, leading to lower risk estimates than the linear model would project. (Munro and Krewski 1981)

No single mathematical procedure is recognized as the most appropriate for low-dose extrapolation in carcinogenesis. When relevant biological evidence on mechanism of action exists, the models or procedures employed should be consistent with the evidence. When data and information are limited, however, and when much uncertainty exists regarding the mechanism of carcinogenic activity, models or procedures which incorporate low-dose linearity are preferred when compatible with the limited information . . .

It should be emphasized that the linearized multistage procedure leads to a plausible upper limit to the risk that is consistent with some proposed mechanisms of carcinogenesis. Such an estimate, however, does not necessarily give a realistic prediction of risk. The true value of the risk is unknown, and may be as low as zero . . . (US Office of Science and Technology Policy 1985)

It is apparent that the choice of mathematical models to represent dose–response relationships involves a substantial element of scientific judgement. Although several models are available, all are subject to criticism. Empirically, several different models can be fitted to most data sets, and it is unlikely that further experimentation, even with large groups of animals, will decisively discriminate between possible models. On theoretical grounds, each model has certain desirable features and limitations. The multistage model has good flexibility to fit a wide range of empirical data and has a reasonable biological basis. However, it, too, may not be optimal in all circumstances.

Within this background of scientific uncertainty, the following conclusions appear to be reasonable guidelines for dose–response assessment.

It is not appropriate to apply the concept of 'thresholds' to carcinogenesis unless dose–response data are available that are inconsistent with a non-threshold model.

The effect of a carcinogen can generally be assumed to be additive to that of ongoing processes or other agents that give rise to 'background' incidence of cancer. Exceptions to this general assumption are appropriate when the carcinogen under discussion can be shown to operate by a mechanism that is distinct from those leading to background incidence or to act synergistically with other carcinogenic exposures.

The current knowledge of the mechanisms of carcinogenic action provides little guidance as to the appropriate choice of models. Although the assumption of low-dose linearity is most generally accepted for carcinogens that interact directly with DNA, dose additivity will lead to low-dose linearity for carcinogens that act at any stage. (California Department of Health Services 1986)

Feedback

The shape of the dose–response curve at low doses is uncertain. There is no universally accepted model for the shape at low doses and scientific judgement is needed in each case. Where there is little information to go on, the LNT hypothesis is normally preferred, but may over-state risk in some cases.

 Activity 5.5

In reading the following guidance from the WHO (1987) regarding exposures to nitrogen dioxide and to nickel in the atmosphere, think about the forms of the two pieces of guidance and consider why they are different.

 Exposure guidelines

Nitrogen dioxide levels of $400\,\mu g/m^3$ and $150\,\mu g/m^3$ are recommended as 1-hour and 24-hour guidelines respectively. The 1-hour guideline is based on the judgement that the lowest-observed-effect-level (LOEL) in asthmatics ($560\,\mu g/m^3$) is not necessarily adverse and a guideline somewhat lower provides a further margin of protection. The 24-hour guideline is based on the judgement that repeated exposures approaching the minimum repetitively observed effect level are to be avoided, so as to create a margin of protection against chronic effects.

At an air nickel dust concentration of $1\,\mu g/m^3$, a conservative estimate of lifetime risk is 4×10^{-4}.

 Feedback

The WHO has taken nitrogen dioxide to be a compound without carcinogenic effects, in which case the guideline was derived from knowledge of the LOAL, LOAEL or NOAEL and application of a protection (safety) factor. For nickel, this has been put through the WHO's two-step procedure which, first, assesses whether the compound is a proven human carcinogen (a group 1 compound); a probable human carcinogen (a group 2a compound has limited evidence of human carcinogenicity and sufficient evidence of animal carcinogenicity; group 2b has inadequate evidence of human carcinogenicity and sufficient evidence of animal carcinogenicity); or unclassified (group 3). Second, having identified it as a potential human carcinogen, epidemiological and toxicological data have been used to identify a risk factor since no absolutely safe level can be defined. The risk factor, which is expressed as the lifetime risk of developing cancer as a result of continuous exposure at the specified level, should be seen as a rough estimate and not the true cancer risk. It serves as a basis for policy makers in balancing risks and benefits and establishing the degree of urgency of the associated public health problem.

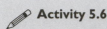 **Activity 5.6**

For the policy maker there are important issues embedded in the choice of a threshold or non-threshold approach for controlling exposures. In reading the following extract from the Commonwealth of Australia (2002), make a note of the answers to these questions:

1 What are the advantages of the threshold approach?
2 What are the advantages of the non-threshold approach?
3 Why should both approaches be treated with caution?

 Threshold versus non-threshold approaches

The important conceptual distinction between non-threshold methods and those which derive an acceptable exposure from the NOAEL using a safety factor is that the safety factor approach makes no attempt to determine a finite level of risk at low exposures whereas the linear methods do make an estimate of risk at low exposures. The NOAEL is assumed to be the threshold dose for the effect. Both approaches have advantages and disadvantages.

The advantages of the threshold approach are that the NOAEL is relatively easy to determine, and the process is simple to use, easy to understand, and allows the use of expert judgement (in setting safety factors). In the few cases where epidemiological data have become available, the ADIs derived by this method have been validated. Additionally, the approach has been applied seemingly consistently by the WHO in the last three decades in deriving ADIs for pesticides.

Because it provides numerical estimates of risk at all doses, the non-threshold approach, in principle, has the potential advantages of allowing: computation of comparative risks in the sub-experimental range, which may be a useful tool in risk management and communication; potency comparisons between chemical agents at a particular risk level; and estimates of the increased risks if a particular dose is exceeded. It has been argued that risk estimates by this approach approximate those seen in humans in some cases and where there are disparities, they are overestimates of the risks.

Both the threshold and non-threshold methods, however, are likely to be unduly influenced by the selection of doses. The choice of the NOAEL is limited to one of the doses included in the experimental design. The biological no effect dose may occur at this dose or at a dose not included in the study. The closeness with which the selected NOAEL truly reflects the actual no effect dose has an obvious impact on the degree of protectiveness in the derived ADI, PTWI or RfD. Furthermore, the NOAEL is influenced by the biological effects monitored, the number of animals in the test groups, the spontaneous incidence of the adverse effect, and the criteria used to determine when the incidence in a test group exceeds that in the controls.

Additional limitations of the threshold approach include: the NOAEL is often perceived as a biological threshold, whereas it is a threshold limited by the experimental protocol; risk is expressed as a fraction of the guidance dose (e.g. ADI); it makes limited use of the dose–response slope; the choice of safety factors has been arbitrary to some extent and the process does not generate a range of estimates of risk, but rather a single estimate of a dose below which no adverse effects are likely to be produced . . .

Non-threshold models currently in use are inflexible and generally do not take account of the complexities of the events between exposure to an agent and the induction of a neoplasm. Risks estimated at doses below the range of experimental data can vary considerably depending on the model used, even though the various mathematical models used generally fit the experimental data equally well. The numerical estimate of the level of risk falsely gives the impression that it represents an exact measure of actual risk. The numerical expression provides little or no information on the uncertainties related to the estimated level of risk, nor does it allow comparison with values for non-cancer health effects.

↻ Feedback

1 Advantages are the simplicity of the approach and the gradually increasing evidence of validity. The approach also allows a consistent approach to the specification of ADIs.

2 Risks at low doses can be estimated and this may help policy makers. There is also some evidence of validity of estimates, and some that they are conservative, i.e. more protective than the model suggests.

3 In toxicity tests on animals, the choice of experimental design parameters influences the NOAEL and hence the ADI, PTWI or RfD, and safety factors remain rather arbitrary. For both threshold and non-threshold models, the uncertainties associated with the predictions are potentially quite large and the numbers quoted should not be taken as strict safety levels or as accurate risk factors.

Summary

The determination of dose–response relationships is an integral part of environmental health risk assessment. So far as environmental toxins are concerned, it is important to distinguish between threshold and non-threshold agents. The type of agent you are dealing with determines the approach to setting an acceptable level of exposure. Whichever type of agent you are concerned with, it is important to be aware of the limitations of dose–response assessments. Despite these limitations, you should ask yourself where we would be without the assessments. The answer is, in an even more uncertain world where policy setting would be yet more difficult.

References

California Department of Health Services (1986) *Guidelines for the Assessment of Carcinogenic Substances*. Sacramento, CA: CDHS.

Commonwealth of Australia (2002) *Environmental Health Risk Assessment: Guidelines for Assessing Human Health Risks from Environmental Hazards*. Canberra: Commonwealth of Australia.

Munro IC and Krewski DR (1981) Risk assessment and regulatory decision-making. *Food Cosmet. Toxicol.* 19: 549–60.

Office of Science and Technology Policy (1985) Chemical carcinogens: a review of the science and its associated principles. *Federal Register* 50(50): 10372–442.

Paustenbach DJ (1989) *The Risk Assessment of Environmental Hazards*. New York: John Wiley & Sons, Ltd.

World Health Organization (1987) *Air Quality Guidelines for Europe*. Copenhagen: WHO.

6 Exposure assessment

Overview

The next stage in the process of quantitative risk assessment is exposure assessment. Exposure assessment is just as important as hazard identification and dose–response assessment. This is logical because if there is no exposure to a hazard, then its existence is unimportant. Here you will learn about the different routes through which exposure may occur and how to quantify them.

Learning objectives

By the end of this chapter, you will be better able to:

- **describe how the body is exposed to environmental chemicals**
- **discuss techniques for determining human exposure to environmental chemicals**
- **distinguish between exposure and dose**
- **calculate exposures and doses.**

Key terms

Bioaccumulation A process that results in the concentration of particular substances being higher in some organisms than in their surrounding environment.

Dose A stated quantity or concentration of a substance to which an organism is exposed over either a continuous or an intermittent period; most commonly measured in units of milligrams per kilogram of body weight of the receiver (mg/kg bw).

Environmental medium A specific part of the environment such as air, water or soil, sometimes referred to as an environmental compartment.

Exposure The degree to which a person is subject to a given risk factor.

Exposure route How an agent enters the body (such as by inhalation, ingestion, contact).

Introduction to exposure assessment

You read in Chapter 3 that exposure assessment is the process of measuring or estimating the intensity, frequency, and duration of exposure of the human population to risk agents. Exposure can occur in a number of ways, such as through ingestion (e.g. drinking water contaminated with arsenic, or consuming food with pesticide residues), inhalation (e.g. inhaling fumes from cooking stoves), and dermal contact (e.g. handling chemicals or contaminated materials).

The most accurate way of assessing exposure is by measuring the concentration of the agent of concern in relation to the presence and activities of affected persons. Measurement, however, is often expensive and may be impractical. It is therefore common to rely upon mathematical models that estimate concentrations to which persons are exposed. Whichever method is used, it is still necessary to approximate the dose.

 Activity 6.1

In their book, *Risk Assessment Methods: Approaches for Assessing Health and Environmental Risks* (1993) Vincent Covello and Miley Merkhofer describe difficulties posed in the assessment of exposures. As you read the following abridged extract, consider the following questions:

1 Why is human exposure assessment difficult?
2 Why is it important to find out who is exposed?

 Exposure assessment

For many risk assessments, exposure assessment is the most difficult task. The reason for this is that exposure assessment often depends on factors that are hard to estimate and for which there are few data. Critical information on the conditions of exposure is often lacking; for example, although industries are generally required to keep records on work-ers' exposures to toxic chemicals, the levels of exposure and the particular chemicals involved are often not known or not recorded. Exposures to the general population are even less well documented due to the limited availability of systems capable of carrying out such measurements.

A major source of complexity in exposure assessment is the strong influence that indi-vidual personal habits can have on human exposure. In the case of food contaminated with risk agents, food storage practices, food preparation, and dietary habits have a major influence on the amount of the risk agent actually consumed. For example, if raw meats have been contaminated with pathogenic micro-organisms, a critical factor in predicting health consequences is whether and to what extent the meat is cooked. As another example, to estimate consumer exposure to a pesticide requires data on pesticide resi-dues, data on how many pesticide-treated food products are consumed by an average person, and data on how many people consume unusual amounts of the pesticide-treated food products.

If the risk agent is encountered through the use of a consumer product, the patterns of use will affect exposure. A solvent whose vapour is potentially toxic, for example, may be used outdoors or in a confined, poorly ventilated living space. Thus, for consumer products, risk assessments need to consider how products will be used.

If exposure occurs through air or water, exposure assessment must consider how the risk agent moves from its source and if it is altered over time. Chemical agents are generally diluted in the environment and may degrade after release. The aim of exposure assessment in this case is to determine the concentration of toxic materials where they interface with target populations.

Another important aspect of exposure assessment is determining which groups in the population may be exposed to a risk agent; some subgroups may be especially susceptible to adverse health effects. These include pregnant women, very young and very old people, and people with impaired health.

Exposure to multiple risk agents often results in portions of the population becoming more sensitive to single agents. Exposure to risk agents that act synergistically greatly complicates risk assessment. Exposure to both cigarette smoke and asbestos results in a rate of cancer incidence much greater than that indicated by the dose–response data for the individual substances. Synergisms also often necessitate that exposure assessment consider the activities in which the exposed individuals engage. Strenuous activity often increases the uptake of risk agents. Multiple sources also complicate exposure assessments. An individual can be exposed to a single risk agent from several distinct sources. Exposure to lead, for example, can come from breathing air, eating food, and drinking water.

 Feedback

1 There is a general lack of exposure data and it is also hard to gather. People are constantly moving around and have widely differing habits. When it comes to exposure assessment, it is frequently the case that 'the devil is in the detail'.

2 For a specific agent, different subgroups may be more or less vulnerable depending upon their personal habits, needs, lifestyle, gender and state of development.

Pathways of human exposure

The primary routes of exposure to environmental risk agents for human beings are through the inhalation of gases, vapours and dusts; through ingestion of foods, water, or unintentionally of other materials including dust and soil; and via skin contact.

 Activity 6.2

Polychlorinated biphenyls (PCBs) constitute a class of 209 man-made, closely related organic chemicals. Previously manufactured in many industrial countries for use in electrical equipment, PCBs are now strictly controlled. A small number have been found to have toxicological effects, but the main concern is that PCBs have been found to have spread throughout the environment where, due to their slow rate of degradation, they are very persistent.

Think about the pathways by which PCBs could spread through the environment to human beings. Then compare them with the feedback below.

Feedback

Figure 6.1 illustrates how chemical agents may spread through the environment from a source and come into contact with people. PCBs in particular can escape from manufacturing plant in the liquid or vapour phase. They also leak from electrical devices during use and following disposal, unless incinerated under carefully controlled conditions. They are soluble in lipid-rich (fatty) tissues and secretions including mothers' milk. PCBs wash into water courses and the oceans, bioaccumulating, because of their fat solubility, in fish, thus entering the food chain. Other routes, affecting land animals, are also active, such as deposition on grass and contamination of animal feed. Today the main source for humans is the consumption of fatty foods such as meat, fish, eggs, milk and milk products, including human milk.

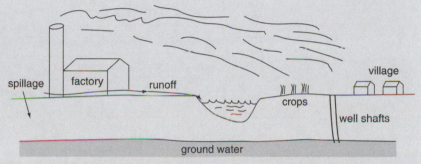

Figure 6.1 Chemical agents may spread from a factory via atmospheric emissions, spillages which contaminate runoff and ground water, tracking out on vehicle tyres, or via shoes and personal clothing. Resulting exposures can be through ingestion, inhalation, and dermal contact with contaminated dusts deposited on surfaces or soil.

Activity 6.3

At one time tetraethyl lead was widely used as a petrol additive for the purpose of improving the fuel economy of cars. This, however, resulted in contamination of the atmosphere by lead, and especially for people living in towns and cities, their blood–lead concentrations were increased following inhalation of lead particles. This resulted in health concerns, because lead exposure is linked with effects on the central nervous system, especially in children. Consequently, many countries have now taken measures to reduce or eliminate the use of tetraethyl lead.

Draw up a list of routes by which people may be exposed to lead emissions from car exhausts.

↻ **Feedback**

Figure 6.2 shows how lead not only enters the body through the lungs but via other media. Pathways include deposition on leafy foodstuffs, deposition on soil and uptake by root crops, and ingestion of trace amounts of contaminated soil or deposited dust via the hand-to-mouth route.

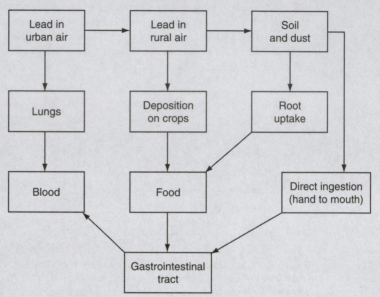

Figure 6.2 Pathways by which lead emissions from vehicle exhausts may contribute to the concentration of lead in the blood of exposed persons

Approaches to exposure assessment

Figure 6.3 provides an overview of the methods available for assessing exposure, both direct and indirect.

Direct monitoring

In this approach individuals carry personal devices which monitor the environment around them. Doctors and nurses who work in a radiodiagnostic or radiotherapeutic capacity in hospitals often wear film badges that record their exposure to ionizing radiation. These badges can be checked periodically to assess exposure. The approach has been extended in recent years through the invention of small, portable devices, known as personal samplers. These can measure a range of atmospheric pollutants.

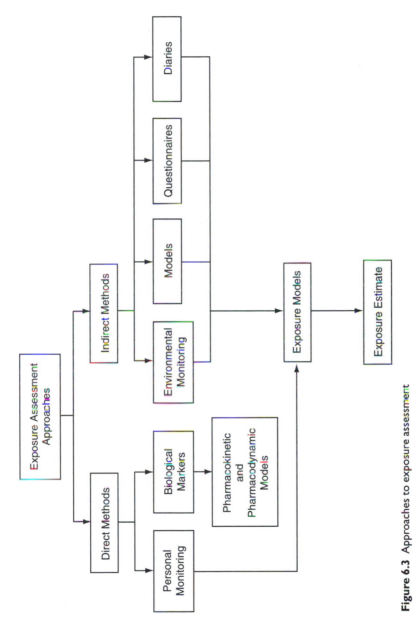

Figure 6.3 Approaches to exposure assessment

Source: Adapted from National Academy of Sciences (1991)

Indirect monitoring

In this approach it is customary to rely upon information from any national, urban or rural monitoring which has been carried out. A good number of countries now have permanent monitoring systems in place which measure air and water quality on a continuous basis at a network of fixed monitoring sites.

Use of biomarkers

Exposure to certain compounds may result in an accumulation of that compound in the body, or it may generate other biochemical or physiological responses which can be measured. Exposure to lead, for example, results in short-term elevated concentrations of lead in the blood. Over the long term, lead will accumulate in hair, teeth and bone and lead levels in appropriate samples can therefore be used to assess cumulative exposure.

Exposure to risk agents may also be measured through indirect biomarkers of exposure. For example, exposure to inorganic lead generates an enzyme known as Delta-ALAD. It is possible to infer exposure to inorganic lead by measuring Delta-ALAD activity in the blood. Table 6.1 lists a number of substances, exposure to which may be detected by suitable biological monitoring.

By inference

In many situations, monitoring data will not exist. In these cases published data from situations which reflect as closely as possible the circumstances of concern may have to suffice.

By modelling

Literally hundreds of models, which are basically mathematical simulations of the real world, have been developed as an aid in predicting exposure. The main group is concerned with describing how specific pollutants, chemical or biological, move from their source through the different compartments (air, water, soil) of the environment. Models are often designed for a specific purpose, for example, to predict the exposure of people living downstream of a plant discharging waste into a river. Table 6.2 indicates the range of models available and their purposes.

As an illustration, Figure 6.4 shows an example of one type of model that is widely available. In the example chosen, the model would take as input the rate of pollution of specified kind emitted from the chimney and compute the concentrations in the atmosphere at some downwind distance. To do this the model needs to know the meteorological conditions at the site (wind speed, direction, air temperature, atmospheric stability) and also the form of the land (whether it is flat or hilly, inland or by the sea).

The outputs of these models are expressed in different units depending upon the medium which is being considered (see Table 6.3).

Table 6.1 Exposure to some substances can be detected by biological monitoring of exposed persons

Substance	Where monitored	Comments
Lead	Blood, tooth, hair	Substantial data are available on the level of risk associated with blood lead ranges. Tooth and hair concentrations measure longer-term, chronic, exposure
Arsenic	Urine	The retention time is short and measurements must be made close to the time of exposure
Mercury	Blood, urine	At equilibrium the concentration of mercury in blood reflects daily intake and is probably the best measure
Cadmium	Urine, blood	Urinary levels tend to reflect body burden whereas blood levels reflect recent exposure
PCBs	Blood and adipose (fat) tissue	Because of the long retention time in fat, long-term exposures are measured
Organochlorine pesticides (aldrin, dieldrin, chlordane, heptachlor, etc.)	Blood and adipose tissue	Because of the long retention time in fat, long-term exposures are measured
Organophosphorus compounds (malathion, chlorpyrifos, etc.)	Blood	By measuring cholinesterase levels

Source: Based on Langley (1991)

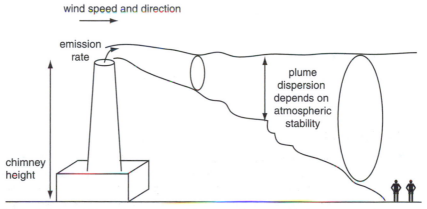

Figure 6.4 Atmospheric dispersion models are simple in principle. They estimate how much a plume of contaminant spreads out and dilutes before it reaches the population.

Table 6.2 Types of model, of varying complexity, available for exposure assessment

Type of model	Typical inputs	Typical outputs
Atmospheric dispersion	Emission rate of specified pollutants; emission characteristics (e.g. height above ground); meteorological data; land topography	Atmospheric concentrations at locations of interest
Surface-water models	Emission rates from local or dispersed sources; flow characteristics of receiving waters; properties of the contaminant (e.g. solubility)	Average concentration as a function of distance from source
Ground-water models	Infiltration rates; local geology; flow pattern; chemistry	Concentration of pollutants in water used for irrigation and consumption
Food chain models	Input rates; empirically derived bioaccumulation rates for relevant organisms	Concentration in food products for human consumption

Table 6.3 Examples of typical measurement units for describing pollutant concentrations

Medium	Measure	Typical units of measurement
Air	Weight of pollutant per unit volume or mass of air	$\mu g/m^3$ (micrograms per cubic metre) ppm or ppb (parts per million or parts per billion by weight)
Air	Volume of pollutant per unit volume of air	ppm or ppb (parts per million or billion by volume)
Water	Weight of pollutant per unit volume or mass of water	mg/l (milligrams per litre) ppm (parts per million by weight)
Soil	Weight of pollutant per unit weight of soil	mg/kg (milligrams per kilogram) ppm (parts per million by weight)
Food	Weight of contaminant per unit weight of food	mg/kg (milligrams per kilogram) ppm (parts per million by weight)

 Activity 6.4

In selecting a model, what kind of factors would you consider?

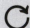 **Feedback**

You would need to consider all or some of the following: the medium through which the pollutant is being transmitted (air, surface water, ground water, etc.); what the characteristics of the source of the pollutant are (continuous or intermittent releases; well-defined point location or dispersed source); what the geographic scale of the problem is (local, regional, national or global); the nature of the vulnerable receptors (humans, animals, plants, or habitats); whether the interest is the population-averaged exposure or specific sub-populations of concern; exposure routes (ingestion, inhalation, dermal contact); and the time frame (retrospective, current or prospective exposures; acute or chronic exposures).

Dose estimation

Estimating contaminant concentrations in the media to which people are exposed is only part of the story of exposure assessment. Models simply tell you about the concentration of the pollutant at the location of the receptor persons. This information must still be converted into the doses actually received by individuals. To do this, you need other kinds of model, sometimes called exposure route models. Exposure route models perform the task of estimating an individual's pollutant intake. This is in principle straightforward. You take the average concentration in the medium (air, water, soil, food) to which the person is exposed and multiply it by the period of exposure and the rate of intake of that medium. For example, if the medium were drinking water, you would need to know the rate of consumption in, say, litres per day, to calculate the dose.

The general formula for estimating chemical intake is as follows (Covello and Merkhofer 1993):

$$I = (C \times CR \times EF \times EP)/BW$$

where: I   = intake (mg/kg of body weight)

       C   = average concentration in the medium during the exposure period

       CR = the amount of air/water/soil/food contacted per unit of time or event

       EF   = exposure frequency (days per year)

       EP   = exposure period (years)

       BW = body weight (kg)

Note that intakes are normally expressed in terms of some quantity, which may be measured in milligrams or micrograms *per kg-body weight*. This is because harmful effects are usually inversely related to body weight, that is, if you have a small body weight, as in an infant, the same dose will do more harm than it would to an adult. However, there is another complication. The above formula estimates *intake*. This may well differ from *uptake*, which is usually the more important parameter. For example, some contaminants will pass quickly through the body and be excreted, or may be exhaled immediately.

In order to use the above formula it is necessary to have data on CR, the contact rate. Since the primary exposure routes are from inhalation of gases, vapours and dusts, and ingestion of contaminated foods, water, soil or dust, much work has been carried out to measure these parameters.

Activity 6.5

In the case of the inhalation of contaminants, it is necessary to know typical respiratory rates. However, respiratory rates are not constant. What are the main factors influencing respiratory rate?

 Feedback

Respiratory rate is affected by age, gender and level of activity. Table 6.4 gives some typical values, measured in litres of air per minute.

Table 6.4 Breathing rates by age, gender and activity level

	Adult male	Adult female	Child (10 years)	Infant (1 year)
Resting (litres/ minute)	7.5	6.0	4.8	1.5
Light activity (litres/ minute)	20.0	19.0	13.0	4.2

Source: Based on Snyder (1975)

In the case of exposure resulting from ingestion of food, liquids, dust or soil, it is necessary to have average consumption data. Food consumption rates have been measured in many countries and standard values have been adopted for some, but clearly these will vary substantially depending upon cultural preferences, availability and income.

In the case of water consumption, typical values are often taken to be 2L/day for adults (70 kg) and 1L/day for children (10 kg). In areas where the ground is contaminated, the primary intake mechanism is often the direct ingestion of contaminated soil or, if atmospheric deposition is the mechanism giving rise to contamination, dust. The view is that pre-school children are most vulnerable to this exposure route. Paustenbach (1989) has reviewed soil uptake studies and has concluded that the amount of soil uptake by a typical child (aged 2 to 6 years) is in the region of 50 or 100 mg/day.

Dermal absorption through contact with contaminated media is harder to estimate. This is influenced by contaminant concentration, the nature of the contaminated medium (solid, liquid, vapour or gas), area of skin exposed, exposure duration, and the dermal absorption coefficient. Specific details of exposure circumstances would be required before intake by this mechanism could be estimated.

 Activity 6.6

Estimate the total uptake in µg/day of lead for adults and children (1–5 years) from simultaneous exposure to lead in air, food and water. Make the following assumptions: the mean lead in air concentration is 2 µg/m³; adults inhale 20 m³/day and children 5 m³/

day of air; the respiratory absorption rate for adults and children is 40 per cent; adults have an intake of 100 µg/day of lead from food with an absorption rate of 10 per cent; children have a lead intake from food of 50 µl/day with an absorption rate of 50 per cent; the water concentration is 25 µg/litre; adults consume 1 litre/day of water with an absorption rate of 10 per cent; children consume 0.5 litre/day with an absorption rate of 50 per cent.

Feedback

For adults, uptake is given by:

$$(2 \text{ µg/day} \times 20 \text{ m}^3/\text{day} \times 0.4) + (100 \times 0.10) + (25 \text{ µg/l} \times 1 \text{ l/day} \times 0.10) = 28.5 \text{ µg/day}$$

For children, uptake is given by:

$$(2 \text{ µg/day} \times 5 \text{ m}^3/\text{day} \times 0.4) + (50 \times 0.50) + (25 \text{ µg/l} \times 0.5 \text{ l/day} \times 0.50) = 35.25 \text{ µg/day}$$

Activity 6.7

Read the following passage from Rodricks (1994) and then, using the adult and child uptake rates for lead calculated above, and assuming adults weigh 70 kg and the children weigh 15 kg, calculate and comment upon the doses of lead received by adults and children.

Calculating dose

Everyone is generally familiar with the term dose, or dosage, as it is used to describe the use of medicines. A single tablet of regular strength aspirin typically contains 325 milligrams of the drug. An adult takes four tablets in one day, by mouth. The total *weight* of aspirin ingested on that day is 1300 mg, or 1.3 grams. But weight is not dose. For reasons relating to how aspirin affects the body biologically, i.e., how it relieves pain, the critical measure is the amount taken into the body divided by the weight of the person, expressed in kilograms. The aspirin *dose* for a 65 kg adult is thus 1300 mg/65 kg = 20 mg/kg body weight (b.w.). The time over which the drug was taken is also important in judging its effectiveness. Our adult took four tablets in one day, and the day is the usual time of interest. So a more complete description of the aspirin dose in this case is given by 20 mg/kg b.w./day. The typical dose units are thus milligrams of chemical per kilogram of body weight per day.

Note – and this is quite important – that if a 20 kg child were to take the same four tablets on one day, his dose would be more than three times that of the adult, as follows: 1300 mg aspirin/20 kg b.w. = 65 mg/kg b.w./day. For the same intake of aspirin, the lighter person receives the greater dose.

Feedback

The dose of lead received by the adults is (28.5 µg/day)/70 kg = 0.41 µg/kg b.w./day, and by the children is (35.25 µg/day)/15 kg = 2.4 µg/kg b.w./day. The implication is that the children receive a dose six times higher than the adults. However, one needs to be careful about the nature of the effects being considered. In the case of sub-acute lead exposure, the primary concern in children is cumulative effects on the central nervous system. In this case, the important parameter may be the long-term average daily uptake.

 Activity 6.8

A more straightforward application of the dose concept is as follows. Consider environmental exposure via ground water which has become contaminated by a widely used degreasing solvent known as trichloroethylene (TCE) of children and adults who get their drinking water from wells. Suppose that the water has been found to contain 1 μg/L (equivalent to 0.001 mg/L), and from that estimate the respective doses. Note: use data given earlier in this chapter.

 Feedback

You need to know that typically adults consume 2 L/day and children 1 L/day of water unless you have more specific information. Also assume, in the absence of specific information, that the adults weigh 70 kg and the children 15 kg. For adults, the daily dose will be: ((1 μg/L) × 2)/70 = 0.00003 mg/kg b.w./day, and for children it will be: ((1 μg/L) × 1)/15 = 0.000067 mg/kg b.w./day. In this case, the children are getting roughly twice the dose of the adults despite consuming half the quantity of water.

Comparing doses with the NOAEL

Environmental health advisers and risk assessors may wish to compare an individual's uptake of environmental chemicals with doses that have been linked to adverse effects in humans. This is often achieved by calculating the maximum daily dose (MDD) or the lifetime average daily dose (LADD) resulting from the exposure, usually in units of mg/kg b.w./day. For chemicals with acute effects, the MDD is usually compared with the NOAEL from short-term animal studies, and for chemicals with carcinogenic potential in long-term bioassays, the LADD is generally compared with the NOAEL identified in long-term tests (Paustenbach 1989). The ratio of the NOAEL to MDD or LADD is then referred to as the *margin of safety*.

What happens to chemicals in the body?

To complete this chapter you should learn something of the fate of chemicals entering the human body. As you have already seen, chemicals may be inhaled through the nose and mouth into the lungs; they may be ingested and swallowed, thus entering the gastrointestinal tract; and they may contact the skin and be adsorbed or absorbed.

As soon as chemicals contact the body, they may damage tissues and cells. They may also enter the bloodstream where they are rapidly circulated around the body, possibly to be transformed (metabolized) by reactions with enzymes, large protein molecules in the cells. The chemicals, or their metabolites, are then excreted in urine, faeces, sweat, and exhaled air. Figure 6.5 illustrates how chemicals may be absorbed, distributed and excreted from the body.

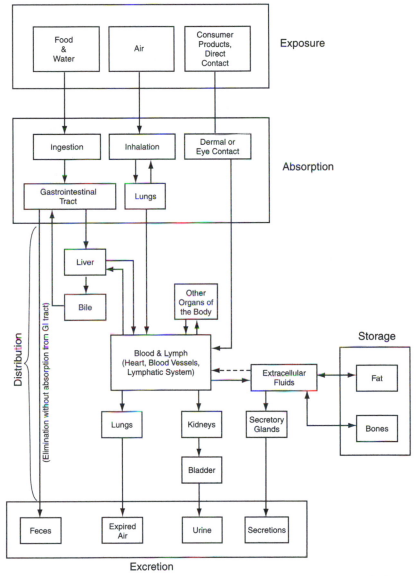

Figure 6.5 Schematic diagram showing how chemicals enter and pass through the body, or are stored

Source: Rodricks (1992)

Summary

Exposure assessment is a crucial component of the environmental risk assessment model yet, because of its complexity, it is often neglected. In conducting a thorough exposure assessment, it may be necessary to consider multiple pathways of exposure and a range of empirical and theoretical techniques are available for determining the importance of these pathways in terms of human exposure. Dose estimation also requires information on human contact with each environmental medium. This in turn depends on body parameters such as breathing rate, food and water consumption, body weight and other characteristics. Standard values have been published by some agencies. These are often helpful but it may be necessary to make allowances if different circumstances apply.

References

Covello VT and Merkhofer MW (1993) *Risk Assessment Methods: Approaches for Assessing Health and Environmental Risks.* New York: Plenum Press.

Langley AJ (1991) Protecting the public: biological monitoring, in El Saadi O and Langley AJ (eds) *The Health Risk Assessment and Management of Contaminated Sites.* Adelaide: South Australia Health Commission.

National Academy of Sciences (1991) *Human Exposure Assessment for Airborne Pollutants.* Washington, DC: National Academy Press.

Paustenbach DJ (1989) *The Risk Assessment of Environmental Hazards.* New York: John Wiley & Sons, Ltd.

Rodricks JV (1994) *Calculated Risks: The Toxicity and Human Health Risks of Chemicals in Our Environment.* Cambridge: Cambridge University Press.

Snyder WS (1975) *Report of the Task Group on Reference Man.* International Commission on Radiological Protection Publication No. 23. New York: Pergamon.

World Health Organization (1987) *Air Quality Guidelines for Europe.* Copenhagen: WHO.

7 | Risk characterization

Overview

Risk characterization is the concluding step in environmental health risk assessment. Its aim is to produce measures of the heath, safety and environmental risks that are being assessed. It requires estimation of the incidence of specified health effects under the various conditions of human or animal exposure described in the exposure assessment and is carried out by combining the exposure and dose–response information. The associated uncertainties of the entire risk assessment process must be included in the description, because the information from risk characterization is used to inform policy makers who need to be aware of uncertainties and any incorporated value judgements when making their decisions.

Learning objectives

By the end of this chapter, you will be better able to:

- **understand the aims of risk characterization**
- **discuss the role, nature and significance of uncertainty**
- **characterize risk.**

Key terms

Conservatism Assuming the worst case in order to err on the side of safety.

Hazard index (HI) The quotient of the maximum daily dose and the acceptable daily intake of a hazardous material.

Unit cancer risk (UCR) An estimate of the excess probability of cancer per unit dose.

Characterizing risks

The aims of risk characterization are:

- to integrate the information from hazard identification, dose–response and exposure assessment;
- to provide an evaluation of the overall quality of the assessment and the degree of confidence which should be assigned to the outputs;
- to describe the risk to individuals, populations and/or the environment in terms of the nature, extent and severity of potential harms;

- to communicate the results clearly and unambiguously to the policy maker;
- to provide information that might be used in communicating with wider interest groups.

Describing risk

Risk may be described in either qualitative or quantitative terms. Qualitative descriptions use terms like 'high', 'medium' or 'low', and, though lacking in numerical precision, can still be useful to decision makers. Figure 7.1 shows a typical scheme for doing this. An important point about this matrix is that it is two-dimensional. This is because risk involves at minimum two components: probability and consequence, either of which can vary from high to low. Sometimes, as you will see in Chapter 8, these are multiplied together to give a single number referred to as an expectation value, but the drawback of this is that information is lost to the policy maker. If you were given such a number (for example, the expected number of deaths per year in your region from avian flu is 100), you would not know if you were dealing with a hazard with rare but potentially large consequences, or a hazard that was regularly having an impact but with lower consequences. However, even though the matrix conveys more information than a single number, it is still a gross simplification and necessarily judgemental in that users have to decide which categories of probability and consequence to assign to the hazards which are of concern to them.

An alternative approach is to express risks quantitatively. There are a number of ways of doing this. The simplest is in terms of 'individual risk'. Individual risk is the probability of a specified individual dying prematurely, or of suffering some other specified harm, as a result of exposure to the hazard. The time period of exposure must be specified. This is often a year (as in the data in Table 3.1), or a lifetime which is usually assumed to be 70 years. Thus, the WHO (1987) states that the

	Consequences			
	Severe	**Moderate**	**Mild**	**Negligible**
Probability				
High	high	high	medium/low	Near zero
Medium	high	medium	low	Near zero
Low	high/medium	medium/low	low	Near zero
Negligible	high/medium/low	medium/low	low	Near zero

Figure 7.1 A simple qualitative matrix for describing environmental risk

Source: UK DoE (1995)

lifetime risk of contracting cancer as a result of being continuously exposed to $1\,\mu g/m^3$ in the air of the human carcinogen vinyl chloride is 1×10^{-6} (1 in a million). In other situations it may be informative to calculate the maximum individual risk. This is the risk experienced by the individual, who may be hypothetical, who is most exposed. Sometimes, for example, it is helpful to calculate the risk to a hypothetical person who lives, eats and works on the immediate boundary of a hazardous area. This represents a worst case scenario. Alternatively, risks may be presented as average individual risks, that is, the individual risk averaged over a population. The data in Table 3.1 show average individual risks associated with common hazards in the UK.

A more sophisticated presentation which is useful in some circumstances is to produce a map of the affected area overlaid with individual risk contours, or in the case of a single point source of risk like a chemical plant, a graph of risk against distance from the plant. Examples of these are shown in Figures 7.2 and 7.3. To produce these figures for a given location, you need information on the distribution of wind directions, speeds and weather types.

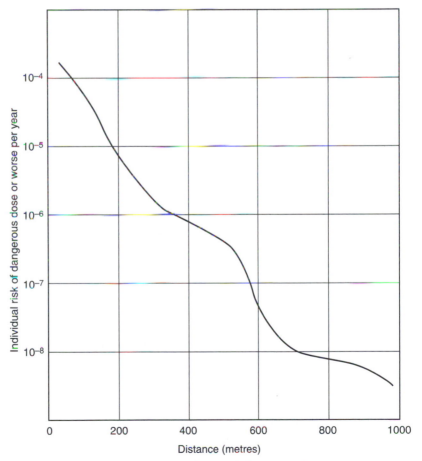

Figure 7.2 Individual risk versus distance downwind of a chemical factory

Source: HSE (1989)

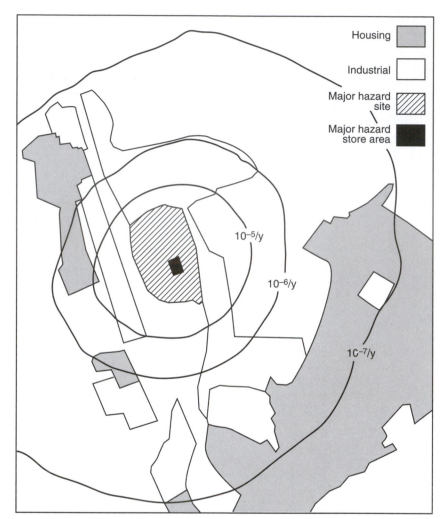

Figure 7.3 Individual risk contours around a chemical factory
Source: HSE (1989)

In carcinogenic risk assessment, a common summary statistic is the upper-bound estimate of the probability of an exposed individual contracting cancer. This is calculated from the product of the lifetime average daily dose (LADD) and the unit cancer risk (UCR). The UCR is an estimate of the excess probability of cancer per unit dose, or, in other words of the carcinogenic potency of the hazardous agent (Covello and Merkhofer 1993). The UCR is determined from the slope of the graph of the dose–response relationship.

For threshold agents, a frequently used summary statistic is the hazard index (HI). The HI is calculated from the maximum daily dose (MDD) received by an individual divided by the estimated acceptable daily intake (ADI). The ADI is usually based on the agent's NOEL or NOAEL combined with the usual safety factors of 10,100 or more as described in Chapter 5.

Being clear about uncertainty

Even when describing risks quantitatively, it must be recognized that doing this with accuracy is seldom feasible because of variability in the hazardous agent and population, and limitations in the toxicological and exposure data. For example, it may be necessary to extrapolate over several orders of magnitude when establishing human health risk factors that are based on animal experiments. A common criticism of quantitative environmental health risk assessments has been that the numbers give a false sense of accuracy and, unless policy makers are warned, may be inadvertently misused.

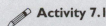 **Activity 7.1**

Read the following excerpt from Paustenbach (1989) and consider why it is important to make assumptions and uncertainties clear when characterizing risks.

 Assumptions and uncertainties when characterizing risks

Although we have come a long way in understanding how we might do a better job in the hazard identification, dose–response assessment, and exposure assessment portions of risk assessment, we have only scratched the surface in our understanding of how to best characterize the risks and how to present them most appropriately to decision makers. If there is any doubt about this claim, one need only read newspaper accounts of the scientific positions of regulatory agencies attempting to characterize the severity of a hazard:

> Excess deaths from lung cancer due to workplace arsenic are down 98%, says the Occupational Safety and Health Administration, based on risk assessment studies. The arsenic standard of OSHA requires engineering controls and other measures to reduce worker exposure from 500 to 10 $\mu g/m^3$. Three risk assessments . . . on the standard's efficacy indicate that excess deaths dropped to 8 to 10 per 1,000 workers from the 375 to 465 per 1,000 that would have occurred under the previous 500 $\mu g/m^3$ standard. (*Chemical Engineering*, 1983)

Among the numerous shortcomings of this news clipping is that the reader is likely to infer that under the 'old' OSHA standard, as many as 46.5% of the worker population were likely to die prematurely due exclusively to occupational exposure to arsenic. In actuality, there was a good deal of discussion within the scientific community whether any increased cancer risk had been observed in epidemiology studies of workers who had been exposed to levels in the vicinity of 500 $\mu g/m^3$. In addition, in an attempt to demonstrate the potential benefits of regulation, much more certainty was attached to the possible results of the regulation than was present in the low-dose extrapolation process. Since the hallmark of a good risk characterization is a thorough description of the range of plausible outcomes, this report would have been more fair had it stated that the old regulation may have posed a risk as great as about 400 in 1,000 and as low as 1 in 1,000,000. As shown here and in most press releases of the past decade, the degree of uncertainty is rarely developed within the risk assessment nor is the significance of the risk communicated in a thorough, easily understood, and objective manner.

Feedback

The news cutting described by Paustenbach, although intended to inform, could clearly be misinterpreted. A difficulty is that news editors generally feel it necessary to present information to their readers in a simple form. The same problem can arise when risk assessors communicate with policy makers. Indeed, policy makers and especially politicians sometimes refuse to accept that uncertainty exists and demand that risk assessors should 'provide unambiguous answers'. However, this is an error – the nature of scientific investigation is being misunderstood and an important policy issue is being sidelined.

 Activity 7.2

What creates uncertainty in risk assessments? From what you have already read about the various stages of risk assessment, make a list of some of the sources that should be taken into account.

 Feedback

One can identify a surprising range of uncertainties associated with each stage of the environmental risk assessment process. The following account lists some, though not all.

Hazard identification stage

- What relative weights should be given to studies (toxicological, epidemiological, etc.) with differing results?
- What statistical significance should be required for results to be considered meaningful?
- What is the significance of a positive finding in a study in which the route of exposure is different from that of the exposed population?
- Should benign and malignant tumours in test animals be counted equally seriously?
- How much weight should be placed on short-term versus longer-term animal tests?
- What additional weight does structural similarity add to the results of toxicological and epidemiological studies?

Dose–response stage

- Which dose–response model should be used to extrapolate from high to low doses?
- For what health effects should dose–response relationships be sought?
- What factors should be used for inter-species conversion of dose from animals to humans?
- How should particular physiological characteristics of an exposed population be accounted for?
- How should information on comparative metabolic rates in animals and humans be used?

Exposure assessment stage

- Which models should be used to predict the dispersion of pollutants through the environment?
- How should dietary habits and other variations in lifestyle be accounted for?
- How could exposure measurements for a small group of people be extrapolated to a population?
- How should exposures of special risk groups, e.g. pregnant women, children, etc., be estimated?
- What is the proper unit of dose?

Risk characterization stage

- What are the statistical uncertainties in estimating the extent of health effects?
- What are the biological uncertainties in estimating the extent of health effects?
- Which dose–response assessments and exposure assessments should be used?
- Which population sub-groups should be the focus of attention?

In general, when estimating risks, there are three broad types of uncertainty to consider. These are:

- uncertainty to do with missing or incomplete information describing the situation under investigation;
- uncertainty affecting a particular parameter, e.g. measurement or sampling errors, variability in the parameter;
- uncertainties in scientific models, e.g. of the dispersion of pollution through an environment, or of the true form of the dose–response function.

While some of these uncertainties could be reduced by the collection of more data, this is not necessarily true and may be prohibitively expensive. Therefore, it may well be necessary to live with the uncertainty. However, various regulatory agencies have produced sets of principles for risk assessment which provide general guidance for alleviating some of the problems of inter-agency inconsistency. Table 7.1 is based on the American experience (Rodricks 1992), but is similar to those in use by other agencies around the world.

✎ Activity 7.3

In looking at the principles in Table 7.1, where do you think the emphasis lies in terms of the protection of health? In particular, note principles 3, 4, 7 and 8.

Table 7.1 Guiding principles for the conduct of environmental health risk assessment

Principle	Guidance
Principle 1	In general, data from studies in humans are preferred to animal data for hazard and dose–response evaluation.
Principle 2	In the absence of human data, or when the available human data are insufficiently quantitative or are insufficiently sensitive to rule out risks, animal data will be used.
Principle 3	In the absence of information to demonstrate that such a decision is incorrect, data from animal species, strain, and sex, showing the greatest sensitivity to a chemical's toxic properties will be selected as the basis for human risk assessment.
Principle 4	Animal toxicity data collected by the same exposure route as that experienced by humans are preferred for risk assessment.
Principle 5	For all toxic effects other than carcinogenicity, a threshold in the dose–response curve is assumed. The lowest NOEL from all available studies is assumed to be the threshold for the groups of subjects (humans or animals) in which toxicity data were collected.
Principle 6	The threshold for the human population is estimated by dividing the NOEL by a safety factor, the size of which depends on the nature and quality of the toxicity data and the characteristics of the human population.
Principle 7	For carcinogens a linear, no-threshold dose–response model is assumed to apply at low doses.
Principle 8	Generally, human exposures and resulting doses and risks are estimated for those members of the population experiencing the highest intensity and rate of contact with the chemical, although other, less exposed sub-groups and people experiencing average exposures will frequently be included.

Source: Rodricks (1992)

 Feedback

These principles are all 'conservative', that is, they all err on the side of caution by assuming the worst case. This can lead to a criticism of risk assessments – that they can result in overly restrictive policies through the application of multiple layers of caution.

The US Environmental Protection Agency (1995) refers to the need for 'an appropriate level of conservatism'. This is an issue you will learn much more about later. Meanwhile, the following principles have been proposed:

 Conservative principles

* actions should adequately protect public health and the environment;
* risk assessments should be transparent;
* conclusions drawn from the evidence should be separate from policy judgements (which are the responsibility of policy makers);

- the nature and likelihood of adverse health effects should be described along with strengths and limitations of the assessment;
- health risk assessment should in many instances be undertaken with a recognition that it is part of a larger environmental assessment;
- to protect public health and the environment an *appropriate* level of conservatism should be incorporated to protect against uncertainties;
- if comparisons are made against environmental health criteria the criteria used should be ones approved by the municipality, region or state;
- when using environmental health criteria to assess a situation, these should preferably be based upon data (toxicological, exposure, etc.) from the region in question.

Summary

You have now examined all stages of the classical environmental health risk assessment model. This may have been quite demanding technically, but it is important, even if you are not technically inclined, to have some understanding of science's contribution to policy. As you have seen, the final stage of risk characterization presents many difficulties for science, involving, as it does, the interface between science and policy. You have seen the importance placed upon the proper presentation of risk assessments as inputs to policy formulation and some of the requirements for dealing with the issues arising. However, environmental health risk assessment is a comparatively new and evolving field and you need to be aware of how it is changing. You will reflect on this in later chapters.

References

Covello VT and Merkhofer MW (1993) *Risk Assessment Methods: Approaches for Assessing Health and Environmental Risks.* New York: Plenum Press.

Health and Safety Executive (1989) *Risk Criteria for Land-Use Planning in the Vicinity of Major Industrial Hazards.* London: HMSO.

Paustenbach DJ (1989) *The Risk Assessment of Environmental Hazards.* New York: John Wiley & Sons, Ltd.

Rodricks JV (1992) *Calculated Risk: The Toxicity and Human Health Risks of Chemicals in Our Environment.* Cambridge: Cambridge University Press.

UK Department of the Environment (1995) *A Guide to Risk Assessment and Risk Management for Environmental Protection.* London: HMSO.

US Environmental Protection Agency (1995) *Guidance for Risk Characterisation.* Washington, DC: US EPA Science Policy Council.

World Health Organization (1987) *Air Quality Guidelines for Europe.* Copenhagen: WHO.

Rational action and environmental health policy

Economic appraisal

Overview

In Section 2 of this book you learnt how environmental health risk assessment is carried out. Section 3 is concerned with risk management, or decision making. Public policy decisions, including those dealing with environmental health, have to reflect economic, social and political realities. You will recall, for example, that the WHO has said that its air quality guidelines 'must be considered in the context of prevailing exposure levels *and* environmental, social, economic and cultural conditions' (WHO 1987). In this first chapter of Section 3 you will consider the role of economics.

Learning objectives

By the end of this chapter, you will be better able to:

- **distinguish between different approaches to environmental pollution control**
- **describe how economic techniques can help environmental health policy makers**
- **understand and question the inputs and outputs of cost–benefit studies of environmental health interventions.**

Key terms

Contingent valuation Survey approach to asking individuals to imagine markets exist and to give their willingness to pay for (accept) benefits (losses).

Ex-ante decisions Decisions that are made in advance of some potential outcome.

Expressed preference studies Studies that elicit consumers' preferences by asking them questions about real or hypothetical scenarios.

Externality Cost or benefit arising from an individual's production or consumption decision which indirectly affects the well-being of others.

Opportunity (economic) cost The value of the next best alternative foregone as a result of the decision made.

Pareto rule An intervention satisfying this rule would improve the well-being of some people without harming anyone else.

Potential Pareto improvement (Kaldor–Hicks principle) The basis for cost–benefit analysis. It stipulates that a reallocation of resources which makes someone better off and someone worse off represents an improvement only as long as those who gain could potentially compensate those who lose.

Quality-Adjusted Life Year (QALY) The value of a year of life adjusted for its quality. A year in perfect health is considered equal to 1.0 QALY.

Revealed preference studies Studies of actual consumer behaviour that indirectly reveal their preferences.

Value of a Statistical Life (VSL) A monetary value used for assessing the efficiency of interventions to improve health or safety of unknown individuals.

Willingness-to-pay (WTP) A method of measuring the value an individual places on reducing the risk of developing a health problem or gaining an improvement in health.

Air pollution in Mexico City – a topical case study

The following case study has been described by Stevens et al. (2005). The Mexico City urban area has an estimated population of 18 million residents. The city is located in a shallow basin and also contains some 3 million vehicles, emitting exhaust which is associated with a number of harmful effects upon the health of its inhabitants. Toxicological and epidemiological studies indicate that the worst of the pollutants emitted by the vehicles is fine particulate matter (PM), similar to soot, which is associated with increased mortality, chronic bronchitis, and other cardio-vascular and respiratory health outcomes. These emissions come mainly from diesel vehicles. Environmental health policy makers have a number of options open to them to deal with this hazard. These include requiring older, smokier, diesel vehicles to be replaced, requiring retrofitting of existing diesel vehicles with either particle filters or oxidation catalysts, or introducing more stringent emission standards for new diesel vehicles.

 Activity 8.1

Given that economics is concerned with the allocation of scarce resources among many needs, what kind of information would you, as a policy maker, wish to have as an aid to choosing which, if any, of the above options to recommend?

 Feedback

It is essential to know how effective each of the measures would be in reducing emissions, exposures, and hence harmful health outcomes. Also important are the costs of the various programmes for the inhabitants of Mexico City, including those of retiring old vehicles, or of purchasing, installing and maintaining filters or catalysts. The policy maker would also need to think about other factors, either costs or benefits, which might result from implementation of these strategies. For example, if it were decided to opt for stringent (and expensive) emission controls on new vehicles, this might encourage owners of older vehicles to keep them on the road for longer. Since older vehicles are generally smokier, this could make things worse. Likewise, if oxidation catalysts were required, would there be any health problems associated with their disposal after they had been used? The policy maker would also want to have some means of comparing the health benefits of each policy option against its costs, and preferably this would be done in the same units of measurement (dollars, pesos, etc.).

Approaches to environmental health protection

It is useful to step back from the above example for a moment and think about the broad categories of approach available to environmental health policy makers. There are three such categories which require some form of regulation, and additionally there are various approaches which rely upon voluntary agreements.

The first and traditional approach can be described as 'design-based command and control', and is one which requires certain technologies or measures to be adopted. For example, these could take the form of a requirement for domestic water suppliers to use a specified filtration system, or to adopt certain management procedures to maintain the system. The second approach is 'performance-based'. This would specify the maximum allowable level of pollution in the medium (air, surface water, drinking water, soil, food, etc.) of concern, as, for example, in WHO air or water quality criteria. A third approach is to use market-oriented techniques. These make use of incentives of some kind or another, for example, taxes or subsidies, to encourage markets to function more efficiently.

 Activity 8.2

All the approaches to regulation described above have advantages and disadvantages. Write down what these might be.

 Feedback

Design-based command and control measures are usually enacted in the form of emission controls. Requiring all polluters to adopt the same controls is fair but potentially wasteful of resources overall, because some polluters may be located far from vulnerable people. Another way of expressing this is to say that the dose, which is what counts, is only indirectly related to the emissions. Performance-based control, on the other hand, which might typically require a polluter to reduce emissions to comply with an environmental quality standard (e.g. the maximum permissible amount of arsenic in drinking water), are fairer from the point of view of those exposed, since nobody should then receive an unacceptable dose of the harmful agent. Another advantage is that the polluter has some flexibility in choosing how to reduce emissions, and may be able to do this at lower cost than if same-for-all, design-based control, were enforced. A disadvantage is that ambient monitoring is required to check compliance and this in itself can be costly. Market-based approaches are more subtle in that they attempt to adjust imbalances in the operation of the market. For example, it may be the case that automobile manufacturers or operators do not feel that ambient air quality is their concern (in economic jargon, it is an 'externality') and so vehicles are designed and operated with little or no attempt to control emissions. However, from the point of view of society as a whole, air is a common 'good' and its quality should be protected. Therefore, a plausible solution is for policy makers to intervene in the market, with subsidies, incentives, or some other measure, so that the externality is internalized in vehicle manufacturers' decision processes. The attractiveness of these types of measures lies mainly in their potential economic efficiency; however, what actually happens remains under the control of the market and not the policy maker.

Table 8.1 includes these three approaches and a number of others to be discussed. Zero or minimum risk is a special case which is applied in circumstances where a hazard is deemed to be intolerable at any level of risk, and examples, based on the actions of some countries, include DDT, PCBs, and the use of lead additives in paint. Risk-based controls, on the other hand, work on the basis that there is a residual level of risk which is acceptable to society, and we will investigate this carefully in Chapters 9 and 10. Utility-based controls, however, are closer to what the remainder of this chapter is about. It should be noted that the word utility has a number of meanings. The common or dictionary definition refers to 'a condition of being useful or profitable'. In Table 8.1, it refers to an approach which weighs both the benefits and the costs of an intervention. In economics, it usually refers to the subjective value, as opposed to the actual value, of something.

Economic appraisal

The example of Mexico City introduced the notion of what is known as economic appraisal. In general, international bodies, governments, municipalities, public and private sector agencies of all sizes, and even individuals, are concerned in one way or another with the economic appraisal of investments of resources including environmental health interventions. That is, all new policies should be subject to comprehensive but proportionate assessment, so as to best promote the public interest.

Management experts in a wide variety of arenas use the 'ROAMEF' cycle to help them make decisions: Rationale → Objectives → Appraisal → Monitoring → Evaluation → Feedback (Figure 8.1).

The aims of economic appraisal are to ensure that all policies, programmes and projects face the following questions before being given the go-ahead:

- Are there better ways to achieve this objective?
- Are there better uses for these resources?

This can be achieved through:

- identifying other possible approaches;
- wherever possible, attributing monetary values to all impacts;
- assessing the costs and benefits of options.

Table 8.1 Summary of alternative environmental control philosophies, all of which can be witnessed in use in the management of environmental hazards

Risk management philosophy	Zero or minimum risk	Ambient standards	Emission standards	Technology-based control	Risk-based control	Utility-based control	Hybrid approaches
Basis	Commitment	Health protection for all	Level playing field for polluters	Use of recognized technology	Scientific simulation	Utility theory	Various
Strengths	Clarity of goal	Compliance relatively easily checked; equity for receptors	Compliance relatively easily checked; equity for emitters	Standardization; encourages technological innovation	Analytical tool; ability to forecast the unknown	Considers both costs and benefits of control	May accommodate equity, utility and other attributes
Limitations	Associated benefits foregone; control costs disregarded	Exposure of receptors not accounted for	Dose and hence harm is only indirectly related to emissions	Potentially expensive; inflexible; may lead to 'ratcheting'	Data hungry; often large uncertainties in e.g. dose–response functions and exposure assessments	Anchored in a particular philosophy; methodological problems, especially in valuing benefits	Difficulty of striking a balance between multiple attributes; requires considerable intellectual input; open to argument
Examples	DDT, PCBs, lead-in-paint	Air quality criteria	Discharge limits to aquatic environment	Use of BAT – best available technology	Control of 'non-threshold' pollutants especially carcinogens	BATNEEC – best available technology not entailing excessive costs	ALARP/ALARA – as low as reasonably practicable/achievable

Source: Ball (2002)

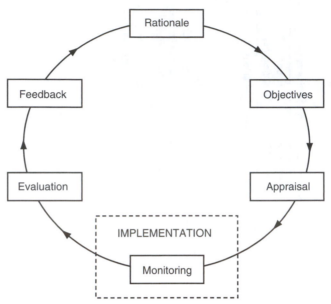

Figure 8.1 This is the 'ROAMEF' cycle, numerous versions of which can be found in management guides

Source: HM Treasury (2003)

Ideally, appraisal is carried out prior to a decision to implement some measure, but it may be used for retrospective analysis of existing policies or measures.

Cost–benefit and cost–effectiveness analysis

Often you will be in a situation where a number of interventions to improve public health are feasible. In this case, the primary tool for appraisal is cost–effectiveness analysis (CEA). You may well have come across CEA, and possibly also cost–benefit analysis (CBA). Of the two main families of appraisal techniques, the techniques of cost–benefit analysis are the most highly developed. There is much more limited experience in the use of a second family of techniques, known as Multi-Criteria Analysis (MCA), though this is growing. MCA techniques are described in Chapter 15. The difference between CEA and CBA is important and you should be able to distinguish between the two.

Imagine that you work for a municipality and your budget provides $10,000 to improve public health. In this case your obvious strategy would be to assess how best to spend this sum in order to bring about the maximum health gain. To do this you might consider different interventions that you could make, how effective they might be, and what they would cost. In this way you could identify the most cost-effective measures and you would implement as many of these as you could until the budget was used up. This would be an example of cost–effectiveness analysis in use.

On the other hand, you might face the different situation of having to bid for resources from an external agency. To do this it might be necessary to demonstrate that the health benefits of the funds, if granted, would warrant the expenditure, i.e. that there would be a reasonable return on the investment in terms of improved health. This would be an example of a cost–benefit (or benefit–cost) analysis (CBA or BCA).

An example of cost–effectiveness analysis

In 1992, the WHO and the Gambian government initiated the National Impregnated Bednet Programme in an attempt to reduce the effect of malaria on the population (Aikins et al. 1998). Local health care centres provided permathrin dipping facilities, an insecticidal treatment, free of charge to local people who brought their bed nets in. The cost–effectiveness of the measure was investigated so that it could be compared with other malaria control measures and other health programmes which were competing for resources.

The main costs were found in insecticide provision, with other costs including administration, transport and facilities. The consequences were measured in terms of reductions in morbidity and mortality, by the effect on school attendance, and by resource savings in the health service and from the point of view of households. Health sector savings were mainly in the form of reduced treatment costs for malaria, but for households there were other benefits besides treatment costs, for example, less time spent caring for sick children.

The results showed that the total programme cost was approximately $90,000, 70 per cent of which was for the insecticide. The estimated number of deaths avoided by the programme was 41, the number of life-years gained was 1,600, and the number of child-years of protection 20,000. Thus, the cost per death voided was $470, per life-year gained $27, and per child-year protected less than $1.

Valuing the costs and benefits of interventions

In general, the relevant costs and benefits of each option (possible intervention) should be assessed. As in the above example, you first have to decide from whose perspective you are carrying out the assessment. The perspective of a national government may differ from that of a private company, a municipality, an NGO, or an individual.

Having decided, you will need to consider all the costs and benefits associated with the intervention. Costs and benefits are normally assessed in terms of market prices. However, in the field of public health you will often be dealing with the costs and benefits of goods that have no market value and if your interest is cost–benefit rather than cost–effectiveness analysis of health interventions, you will have to go a step further and find a means of placing a value on health. The problem is that human health has no market value because it is not a traded commodity, press gangs and slavery having been outlawed, if not eliminated.

Yet another example of a good, or commodity, which is not directly traded is people's personal time. From the point of view of a company you might well include in your cost–benefit assessment the time of your own staff (and price it according to their wages and overheads) but not of other parties, e.g. the public, who might be affected. Thus, time looking after sick children might be excluded, though from a societal perspective it should be considered.

These non-traded goods are sometimes referred to as *externalities*. The problem with externalities is that if they are omitted from the balance sheet, perhaps because they are not seen as capable of being valued, they may not be considered at all in the policy maker's decision process. Later on in this chapter we will consider how to value such non-traded commodities.

Environmental health applications

The fundamental goal of economic decision making is to maximize the individual's well-being by increasing benefits, and to reduce the disbenefits or harm. We are now going to consider, from a theoretical perspective, what this implies in the context of environmental health policy.

In terms of environmental hazards we might be thinking, for example, of harms resulting from exposure to vehicle exhaust fumes in the atmosphere of Mexico City, cadmium contamination in agricultural soil, mercury in the aquatic environment, or exposure to ionizing radiation. In this sense, it is important to realize that maximizing an individual's well-being does not mean minimizing either exposure or risk. This is because, according to economic theory, an individual would seek to maximize his overall benefits and, apart from the harm caused by the exposure, there is also the cost of controlling the exposure to consider. Note that there may also be other side-effects of control interventions which may need to be factored into the decision. For example, the banning of lead additives in petrol, which was a very popular measure in some countries, reduced engine performance and fuel economy, leading to higher emissions of other pollutants. Primarily, however, resources used to control one hazard cannot be put to other beneficial uses and so, in economic terminology, they have an *opportunity cost*.

The crucial implication of this is that there is an optimal level of control, and that this is not normally one which signifies zero risk. Figure 8.2 illustrates this. The horizontal axis measures the level of risk due to the exposure of an individual to some environmental hazard. Risk increases from zero on the left to some value R_1 on the right. On the vertical axis is measured the expected harm in the form of either harm to health or 'harm' in the way of the costs of controlling the risk. The 'control cost' curve in Figure 8.2 shows how the cost of control typically varies as successive interventions are made to reduce exposure to the risk. Interventions may require either hardware or behavioural changes, both of which are deemed to imply a cost. At R_1 it is assumed that there is no control, so the cost of control is zero. As exposure is reduced (moving left from R_1 on the x axis), the control cost curve rises increasingly steeply. This is reasonable because in seeking to control any harmful exposure one would normally go for the least costly and most effective measures first. At the point R_2, the control cost is h_c.

Also shown in Figure 8.2 is the expected harm to health due to this risk exposure. The harm is taken to increase linearly with exposure. This, as you will now be aware, is an assumption, but one which is commonly made in, for example, assessing the health risks of exposure to non-threshold pollutants, as discussed in

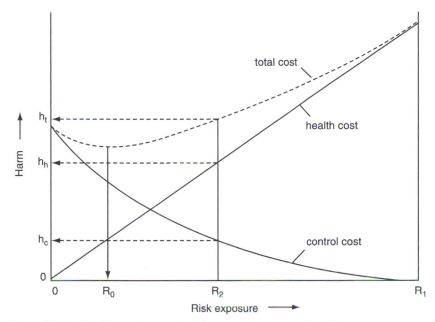

Figure 8.2 Health effects and costs (y axis) versus risk exposure (x axis)

Chapter 5. Recall that this type of dose–response function is referred to as 'the linear no threshold' (LNT) hypothesis because it is a straight line passing through the origin. Thus, at the exposure level R_2, the harm to health is given by h_h, from which the total harm at exposure level R_2 is given by:

$$h_t = h_c + h_h.$$

What is of most interest is the total cost curve, arrived at by adding the appropriate health and control costs for each risk exposure. The most important feature of this total cost curve is that it has a minimum value at a non-zero level of risk exposure, shown as R_0. This is the point at which an individual can be said to have 'optimized' her risk exposure. In practice, there are uncertainties that make identification of the optimal control point more complex, but the principle is the same.

A different situation pertains when determining the appropriate level of, say, environmental control at the population level. This is because control is usually in the form of discharge limits on pollutants or ambient quality standards which have to be optimized for an entire population who individually may have different susceptibilities and needs. In this case we are dealing with public, rather than private, goods and the economic approach is to compare the total benefits for everyone with the total cost, and to choose the level of control that maximizes the difference between total benefits and costs. This approach is based on the concept of the Pareto improvement named after Vilfredo Pareto, an economist (1848–1923) and the Kaldor–Hicks qualification of it.

Pareto defined an improvement as any change that improves the well-being of some people without harming others. Although this seems a logical rule, its application could result in interventions which benefit the well-off while doing nothing for the poor, thus increasing inequality. Another difficulty is that the strict Pareto criterion does not permit interventions which cause a disbenefit to anyone at all. Usually, in the practical world, it is necessary to consider interventions which benefit some people but may harm at least some others. Hence decision makers normally apply the Kaldor–Hicks rule, which says that there is a *potential Pareto improvement* if an intervention creates a situation in which the beneficiaries gain enough that they could, in theory, compensate the losers for their losses. Thus, in order to determine if an intervention offers a potential Pareto improvement, it is sufficient to sum the monetary benefits and losses across the affected population and see if the difference is positive or negative.

 Activity 8.3

Give an example of an environmental health intervention consistent with the strict Pareto criterion and an example of one satisfying the Kaldor–Hicks rule.

 Feedback

If you think about the wider implications of environmental health interventions, including the fact that they require resources to be consumed which constitutes a disbenefit for people who pay for them but who may not receive the benefits, then it is very hard to think of any interventions which satisfy a strict Pareto criterion. Even if you do not consider resource implications, it is usually the case that environmental health interventions will cause some form of disbenefit to some people. The banning of the use of DDT in many countries, for example, would be seen as a benefit by those concerned about the effect this chemical has on the environment, but as a disbenefit by those trying to control malaria. Potentially, however, it might be possible to argue the case for the banning of DDT under the Kaldor–Hicks rule if you could show that the environmental benefits to those who gained were greater than the health losses to those exposed to malarial infection. Whether or not a good case could be made is debatable (Bate 1999a, 1999b).

The ethical debate

The above discussion leads directly to the issue of placing monetary values on non-traded goods, for if techniques such as cost–benefit analysis are to be used, both the costs and the benefits must be valued in monetary terms. For the environmental health policy professional, the non-traded goods are clearly human health, human safety, human lives, and the environment. This is a difficult area on two counts. First, it raises ethical questions about the very practice of putting monetary values on things like human health. Second, if the practice is accepted, there is the question of how you actually arrive at numerical values for the purpose of cost–benefit calculations.

Activity 8.4

The following passage, adapted from Barbara Soby and David Ball (1991), describes arguments against putting monetary values on human health. As you read the extract, think about your own position. Do you agree with the arguments or not? Can you think of counter-arguments?

 How to place a monetary value on human health

There are many arguments against valuing life and health in monetary terms. Some revolve around practicalities of how to do it, but other arguments of a more fundamental nature exist. The objections are as follows:

1　The very thought of placing a value on human life and health is anathema. The argument is that life is priceless and that everything possible should be done, regardless of cost, to save an individual.

2　All lives are not equal. Similarly, all deaths are not equal. Placing the same value on all lives may not therefore be appropriate. For example, one health programme may reduce the risk of a slow, painful death while another would reduce the number of quick sudden deaths. Similarly, not all would agree that saving 20 adult lives is the same as saving 20 children.

3　Economic methodology lacks the sophistication to deal with the many aspects of value in a human life. Therefore, decisions should continue to be made on a case-by-case basis.

4　Even if a value could be placed on a human life, other factors which must be considered in the decision making process remain unquantified, such as epidemics and catastrophes, psychological trauma and the age of victims.

5　In selecting health programmes, society is concerned with more than just getting the biggest health gain for its money. It is concerned with liberty, civil rights, and equity and these ethical considerations cannot be quantified.

 Feedback

The first of the above arguments is outwardly the most problematic. Nobody wants to put a monetary value on human life or someone's health. In fact, however, this is not what is being done when monetary values are assigned to health and life for policy purposes because the values are for use in forward planning (that is, from an ex-ante, position) and importantly involve small changes in health risk. They are in no way meant to measure the intrinsic worth of individuals or their well-being. Soby and Ball (1991) go on to say that since resources for increasing health or safety are limited, placing an explicit value on health can help decision makers make more efficient decisions, thus preventing more ill health and saving more lives. Indeed, every time a decision is made to spend or not to spend on a health prevention measure, human health is implicitly valued. Failure to be explicit about it does not mean that health, life or injury is not being valued, merely that the valuation is hidden. Furthermore, not placing an explicit value on health and life does not provide a neutral stance: instead it potentially undervalues health, or over-values it, leading in both cases to inefficient spending on health.

With respect to the second objection, there is no reason in principle why qualitative weighting factors should not be used to accommodate these issues, although the evidence is that the factors themselves are not greatly different from unity. The remaining three objections address the decision making process, and not the valuation of health *per se*. The objections are legitimate and deserve attention, but do not force one to dismiss the role of health valuation. Instead, a policy maker using such values in policy analysis should retain the option of including these other factors within her decision making model.

 Activity 8.5

The economist Michael Jones-Lee (1984) approaches the ethical dilemma by examining the alternatives to valuing health and concludes that these pose their own ethical problems. In reading his list of four alternatives, consider how these ethical problems arise:

1 Ignore estimates of the value of health on the grounds that there is no obviously correct way to value health or potential loss of life and because it is morally repugnant to try to do so.
2 Use informal judgement and educated good sense to estimate the benefits of health interventions.
3 Set environmental standards (e.g. environmental quality standards or emission standards) to protect health regardless of cost and use those instead.
4 Use cost–effectiveness analysis to identify the option that provides the greatest health gain at least cost.

 Feedback

The first approach effectively places the value of health, and life, at zero or infinity. Either way, this will lead to a loss of efficiency and less good will be done. The second approach, which relies on informal judgement, is likely to be inconsistent and therefore inefficient also. The setting of environmental standards begs the question of the criteria by which the standards are set (as the WHO has said, standards, *inter alia*, have to take account of economics). Finally, cost–effectiveness analysis provides no indication of how much it is reasonable to allocate towards environmental health protection.

From the above discussion you will note that the application of cost–benefit analysis in health-related decision making is not to be casually undertaken. It is rightly an area of considerable sensitivity and the professionals who use it must be able to justify their actions as well as understand the associated limitations of the approach. We now move on to the second major issue, which is how to arrive at valuations of health states, and life even, for use in ex-ante environmental decision making.

Valuing health and valuing safety

If commodities of interest cannot be valued from market data, it is necessary to resort to other techniques developed by economists. Let us start with arguably the most difficult proposition – valuing a human life. Recall that this is attempted for the purpose of ex-ante decision making about health interventions which will reduce risk, in most cases by small amounts, and is not therefore about the intrinsic value of health or life.

In the early days, by which is meant up to some 50 years ago, it was suggested that a monetary value might be assigned to a human life by examining one or more of the following:

- life insurance coverage
- legal compensation
- the Human Capital approach.

Although seeing how much life insurance people purchased is simple enough, this method quickly fell out of use because it was realized that insurance, where it was purchased, was usually for the benefit of a person's heirs and so was not therefore an indication of that person's own valuation of his or her life. Likewise, although it was suggested that court awards for cases involving death and injury might give a guide to the value of avoiding death and injury, this also proved problematic. This was because awards may contain a punitive element, are frequently to compensate surviving family members rather than provide a sum equivalent to the value of the deceased's life, and represent ex-post (after an event has occurred) decisions rather than ex-ante decisions (which is what policy choices are), which may not be the same. Nonetheless, painstaking work by the health economist Ted Miller (1990) in the USA has enabled him to value a human life, by careful use of this technique, at $3m, and this value is widely used in the USA for safety and health decision purposes. Until the mid-1970s the favoured approach in the UK and some other countries was that known as Human Capital. This valuation is based on the loss of expected future earnings of an individual experiencing a fatal or non-fatal accident. The calculation takes account of the average age of individuals at risk, the probability of an accident occurring, and either gross earnings or earnings net of consumption.

As an example, if it is believed that the average age of car drivers who die in road traffic accidents is 40 years, that their future earnings would have averaged $5,000 per year, and that they would have retired from work at 65 years, then what has been lost in terms of earnings is (65 – 40) × $5,000, or $125,000 and this is the value of their life according to the Human Capital approach. While relatively simple, the approach is clearly open to the criticism that the valuation is solely in terms of people's economic output. Unsurprisingly, this came to be seen as too cold-blooded, for people's lives are surely worth more than their wages, and in any case some people are not employed, yet their lives are still valued.

By and large, the preferred techniques for valuing life and non-fatal injuries, at least in Europe, now centre upon a suite of techniques under the banner of willingness-to-pay (WTP). There are many authoritative documents which describe these techniques, but a useful reference which is regularly updated and can be found on the internet, is *The Green Book* of the UK's HM Treasury (2003).

The methodology is as follows: first decide whether the impacts of activities or interventions can be measured and quantified, and if prices can be determined from market data. If this cannot readily be done, use willingness-to-pay (WTP) to value a benefit, where WTP is determined by inferring a price from observing consumer behaviour. If this does not provide values, determine whether WTP can be estimated by asking people what they would be willing to pay for a benefit, or (in the case of a cost) how much compensation consumers would demand in order to accept it.

The approach raises new issues. For example, how could you infer a price or value of something like health by observing consumer behaviour?

Activity 8.6

If you are a householder, how many smoke sensors or other recommended safety devices have you fitted in your home? As many as the manufacturers or the fire brigade recommend? Or did you decide to install just a few (or perhaps none at all) in view of the cost and trouble? Could you infer something about your valuation of your own safety by studying your behaviour in relation to the purchase or non-purchase of safety devices? Think about these questions in your own context and write down some answers.

Feedback

Researchers have studied the purchasing behaviour of consumers in consumer societies with regard to smoke sensors and other items and from this have been able to place limits on the value of life to which consumers appear to be responding. Making these calculations does require some heroic assumptions. One is that consumers understand the risk associated with buying and not buying smoke sensors or other safety devices. Another is that they perform some sort of intuitive mental calculation of the risk of harm in deciding whether to purchase them or not.

Despite these difficulties, numbers have been generated by studies such as these. If you can find the data, the crucial part of the calculation is this: if a consumer is prepared to spend an equivalent of $5 a year on smoke detectors to reduce her risk of dying in a fire by 1 in 50,000 per year, then that consumer's value of her own life for safety purposes is given by:

$$\$5 \div \left(\frac{1}{50\,000}\right) = \$250,000$$

This is because the $5 in effect purchases a fraction of that consumer's life equal to $\frac{1}{50\,000}$. Note that we are talking about a tiny fraction $\left(\frac{1}{50\,000}\right)$ of a person's life, not a whole life, when this calculation is done. These calculations are only valid in such circumstances, not when whole lives, especially of known persons, are at stake.

A second WTP (or, more accurately, willingness-to-accept (WTA)) approach is to study how much workers in risky jobs, such as mining, railway maintenance, deep sea fishing, or sea diving, are paid for their work. It is logical that they should receive extra pay in order to be attracted into or compensated for more dangerous work. Some research suggests that this is the case, and valuations of life based on these 'compensating wage differentials', as they are known, have been derived.

Within the discipline of health economics, the above techniques are known as 'revealed preference' methods. This is because people's valuations of health risks have been revealed by their behaviours, either at home or in the jobs they choose. A related technique is to study how much institutions spend on health and safety programmes. This was touched on when we discussed the work by Tammy Tengs and colleagues in Chapter 2. If you can find out how much institutions are spending on specific health or safety interventions and what that means in terms of greater health or safety, it is relatively straightforward to calculate the implied value of health and safety. For example, if an agency has spent $1 million on a health measure which it is believed will save 50 lives during its period of application, then that agency clearly values a life at $20,000 *or more*.

Figure 8.3 shows the range and type of WTP approaches, from which it can be seen that there is a second type known as 'expressed preference'. These techniques attempt to overcome a key difficulty of revealed preference techniques, that is, that consumers may have other things on their mind when they make their decisions. For example, a homeowner may buy smoke sensors or some other safety measure to protect her children rather than herself, or may not understand the risk and be persuaded more by advertising than any personal calculation of risk and benefit.

The solution to these problems is to pose a hypothetical situation to respondents in the form of a question and ask them to respond. In this way the question can be tailored precisely to address the point in which the researcher is interested. This method is sometimes referred to as 'contingent valuation' because it is contingent upon the existence of the hypothetical situation described.

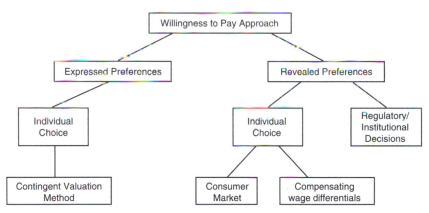

Figure 8.3 The range of WTP approaches available

Source: Ball and Soby (1995)

✎ **Activity 8.7**

Here is an example of a fairly typical expressed preference WTP question. Answer it and see if you can calculate your own value of your life.

Expressed preference WTP

Imagine that you wish to travel by bus from where you live to somewhere else. Imagine that there are two bus companies, A and B, available for you to choose from. The services are identical except for two things. It is known that, and you accept, that buses run by company A are more likely to result in fatal accidents than those run by B. The risk of dying on a journey on a bus from A is $\frac{1}{50\,000}$, whereas on one of B's buses it is one-third of that, i.e. $\frac{1}{150\,000}$. The fare on bus A is $15. The question is, how much more would you be prepared to pay to travel on a bus operated by B company? Having decided that, what then is the implied value of your life?

 Feedback

Logically, you should be prepared to pay something extra for your greater safety. Suppose you are prepared to pay $2 more to go with company B. In effect, this would buy you a risk reduction of:

$$\frac{1}{50\,000} - \frac{1}{150\,000} = \frac{2}{150\,000}$$

That means that for $2 you have avoided a risk of $\frac{2}{150\,000}$ to your life, so the implied value of your life is:

$$\$2 \div \left(\frac{2}{150\,000}\right) = \$150,000$$

Researchers typically obtain answers to these types of WTP questions from randomly selected samples of 1,000 or so people in the population of interest. Zeros, which are not uncommon, and other 'strange' answers would be discarded, and the remaining results essentially averaged (or the median taken) to come up with a representative societal value of an individual's life. Sometimes the values arrived at are supplemented by an estimate of gross lost output (that is, wages not earned as a result of dying prematurely, as in the earlier Human Capital calculation), and any medical and ambulance costs. Table 8.2, for example, shows values from the UK Department of Environment, Transport and the Regions in £(1997) per road casualty, with the second column of data being based on WTP techniques derived from

Table 8.2 Data from the Road Safety Division of DETR

	Lost output	WTP contribution	Medical and ambulance costs	Total (£)
Fatal	294,772	552,252	553	847,577
Serious	12,431	76,654	7,535	96,621
Slight	1,314	5,612	558	7,485

Source: DETR (1997)

a WTP survey using questions similar in style to that in Activity 8.7. The resulting valuation is often referred to as the VSL (Value of a Statistical Life), since it applies not to a particular individual but to an unknown 'statistical person'.

Currently, the UK Department for Transport (DfT) uses a value of £1.145 million per fatal casualty prevented (in year 2000 prices). This is used in the context of road safety investment decisions. DfT also attributes monetary values to the prevention of non-fatal casualties, also based on WTP techniques, as shown in Table 8.2 (http://www.dft.gov.uk). The figure currently used for a serious road injury is £128,650, and for a slight road injury £9,920. Valuations generally increase each year due to changing prosperity, but sometimes they may change because of revisions to the methodology (as when the UK switched from pure Human Capital to WTP in about 1985, causing the valuation of a life to jump from £185,000 to £465,900). Similarly, the UK Health and Safety Executive (2001), whose primary responsibility is occupational health and safety, uses a value of £1 million (2001 prices) for the value of preventing a fatality, and most other UK agencies use similar values.

Around the world many safety valuation studies have been carried out. Figure 8.4 shows how widely the results are scattered. There are different ways of dealing with results such as these. One is to select a middle value by some means and another is to use a range of values. The former is more convenient and is the conventional approach, but the latter is perhaps more realistic – it also forces the user to acknowledge uncertainties.

Valuations of this kind are not restricted to matters of safety in relation to accidents. They are also applied in occupational health and safety, for example. Similar approaches are also found in health care services where it is necessary to consider the cost–benefit ratio of alternative means of investing resources. The main difference in the health sector is that the health impacts, or health conditions being considered, are not simply about saving lives, but about improving quality of life. As a consequence, in the health sector, the term QALY, standing for quality-adjusted life year, is encountered. The QALY scale allows both life years and quality of life to be expressed in a single measure by weighting life years (saved or lost) by the quality of life experienced in those years. QALYs need to be valued too. This can either be done directly by expressed preference WTP studies using different health states as the numerator, or it could be done by linking the train of one's remaining life years, measured in QALY units, to the WTP-derived value of life (Ball and Soby 1995). In the latter case, consideration needs to be given to the issue of discounting, described below.

WTP techniques have also been applied to environmental assets as an aid to environmental decision makers. *The Green Book* (HMT 2003) contains useful examples, which you can follow up if you wish, ranging from the valuation of air quality to landscape, water quality, noise, the cleanliness of bathing beaches and sea water, and the recreational value of forests. Other techniques are available too, for valuing environmental resources. If this attracts your interest, a useful introduction has been written by RK Turner et al. (1994).

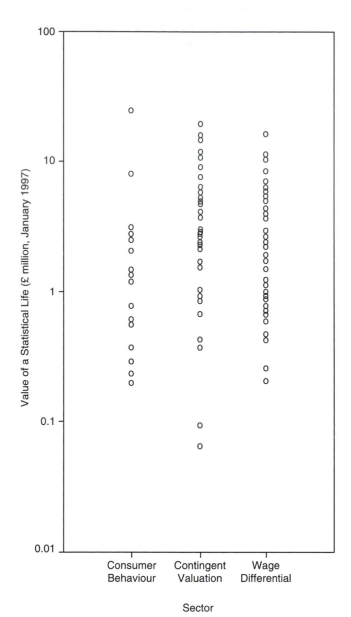

Figure 8.4 The range of values of a statistical life from numerous studies
Source: Ball (2000)

Discounting

Discounting is a sometimes complicated and contentious issue and you can find much about it on the internet. It encompasses the human sentiment that 'A dollar today is worth more to me than a dollar next year', or, with some extension, that 'Happiness is worth more to society now than next year.'

Discounting has come to mean any process of revaluing a future benefit to yield a present value (or value today). The process of discounting reflects the complexities of financial markets, politics, and human interests, but tends to be expressed in fairly simple mathematical terms. Thus, the Present Value of some quantity (PV) is given by:

$$PV = X_t/(1 + r)^t$$

Where X_t is the expected benefit or cost of some item t years in the future and r is the discount rate. The formula implies that having an amount PV in cash now is as good as having a greater amount X_t in cash in t years' time. So if you were told you would receive \$1,000 in ten years' time, and if the discount rate were 5 per cent (i.e. $r = 0.05$), then the present value would be \$613.91.

Using a similar approach, the present value of a future stream of costs and benefits associated with a project or safety intervention can be estimated and compared. The recommended discount rate, sometimes referred to as the Social Time Preference Rate (STPR), is 3.5 per cent in *The Green Book*, although the effect of different rates is tabulated (Annex 6 of *The Green Book*). Generally, the higher a discount rate, the less important appears the future. For this reason lower discount rates are used for projects with lifetimes in excess of about 30 years. For example, for projects extending to more than 300 years a discount rate of 1 per cent is recommended. Even this is contested in some circles, however, as being too high and devaluing the future.

If you need to evaluate projects into the future, then consideration of discounting will be necessary, so follow it up in more detail (e.g. Annex 6 in *The Green Book*) and look at a number of sources for advice. There are standardized procedures to follow but be aware of the arguments for and against. The choice ultimately is political.

Back to Mexico City

This chapter began with a case study of air pollution in Mexico City. The authors of the study (Stevens et al. 2005) were able to estimate the costs of the various programmes to reduce fine particulate emissions from diesel vehicles, and their effectiveness in reducing the concentrations of soot in the air. In turn, by using models, they estimated population exposure under the different programmes and finally, with the aid of suitable dose–response curves, the health benefits of reduced emissions in terms of annual lives saved.

Activity 8.8

One particular problem faced by the authors was that of valuing, in dollars (or some other currency), the value of the health benefits of the resident population. As you read the following edited passage, note the difficulties and how they were approached.

 Deriving a VSL

To compare the health benefits of a retrofit program to its costs, the benefits and costs were converted to a common metric. We assigned monetary values to the reduction in mortality risk using the value of a statistical life (VSL) methodology. VSL is a measure of individuals' willingness to trade wealth for small changes in mortality risk; it is *not* a measure of the intrinsic worth of an individual. Because individuals in developing countries earn less, it follows that they are usually willing to pay less (or accept less compensation) for reductions (or increases) in mortality risk. Therefore, we expect the average Mexican VSL to be lower than the average US VSL.

Ideally, we would derive a VSL from studies in Mexico. However, only one study of VSL is available for Mexico. Given that VSL estimates often vary significantly among studies, we estimated a range by adjusting US estimates of VSL for the difference in income, using an estimate of the income elasticity. The income elasticity of VSL is defined as the proportional difference in VSL associated with a proportional difference in income. Income elasticity observed in developed country analyses is typically less than 1, which indicates that as wealth decreases, the proportion of income an individual is willing to pay to eliminate a specified risk increases. Two studies found an income elasticity of approximately 0.5 when comparing a number of VSL studies in developed countries. In contrast, comparing VSL estimates from middle-income countries (including Mexico) to estimates for high-income countries indicates that income elasticity is much higher, around 2.

A plausible range for a Mexican VSL was obtained by extrapolating from US estimates using income elasticities of 0.5 and 2. Given that the US EPA's central estimate of US VSL of $6.2 million (adjusted to year 2000) and the Mexico/US gross national income per capita ratio of 0.17, the range for Mexican VSL is $170,000 to $2.5 million.

 Feedback

To make a direct comparison of the costs of the interventions against their health benefits it was necessary to value the health benefits in monetary terms. A difficulty is that studies of the value of health and safety have mainly been conducted in higher income countries, so what data could be used? The authors tackle the problem by using the US value of a statistical life (VSL) and scaling it according to the ratio of the gross national per capita income for Mexico and the USA. The calculation takes note of the fact that preferences for spending on health as a function of income in middle income countries may differ from that in high income countries. This is captured by stating the VSL as a range. Note that this is an area of some sensitivity as it may impinge upon national pride if interpreted in a certain way.

Activity 8.9

Read the following abridged passage by Stevens et al. (2005) which summarizes the conclusions of their study on Mexico City, and note how their recommendations are expressed.

 Relevant factors in decision making

Retrofitting diesel vehicles that circulate in Mexico City immediately or in 2010 with any of several technologies that reduce particulate emissions is likely to provide net benefits to society . . .

The results of this analysis are one input that decision-makers should consider when designing policies to improve air quality and public health in Mexico. Other factors that decision-makers will consider include the difficulties associated with implementing a retrofit program, the expected benefits of other policies that reduce emissions and improve public health, and popular demand for policies that improve air quality and public health. While a benefit–cost analysis clarifies the expected outcome of a certain policy, it cannot capture all of the relevant factors that go into a policy decision.

 Feedback

It is important to be aware that cost–benefit studies are generally regarded as an aid to decision makers and not as an alternative. This is because cost–benefit studies, even though they can internalize some quantities which were formerly omitted, do not internalize all conceivable externalities. Depending on how widely the study is framed, there may also be other ways of achieving the desired goal, for example, by encouraging greater reliance upon public transport. In short, CBA studies do not tell policy makers what to do, but they should assist them in their task.

Summary

It is widely accepted that economics has an essential role to play in helping environmental health policy makers decide how best to allocate available resources. Economists have devised a range of techniques for valuing non-traded goods including health, safety and environmental resources. This information permits these items to be quantified alongside the costs of environmental health interventions, so that the efficiency of interventions may be determined. In this chapter you learned how these activities are carried out and applied to environmental decision making.

References

Aikins MK et al. (1998) The Gambian national impregnated bednet programme: costs, consequences and net cost-effectiveness. *Social Science and Medicine* 46(2): 181–91.

Ball DJ (2000) Consumer affairs and the valuation of safety. *Accident Analysis and Prevention* 32: 337–43.

Ball DJ (2002) Environmental risk assessment and the intrusion of bias. *Environment International* 28: 529–44.

Ball DJ and Soby B (1995) Valuing consumer safety. *International Journal for Consumer Safety* 2(3): 117–31.

Bate R (1999a) Pollutants treaty condemns the poor. *Chemistry and Industry*, 1 March, p. 200.

Bate R (1999b) *What Risk? Science, Politics and Public Health*. Oxford: Butterworth-Heinemann.

HM Treasury (2003) *The Green Book: Economic Appraisal and Evaluation in Central Government*. London: The Stationery Office. Also available on the internet.

HSE (2001) *Reducing Risks, Protecting People: HSE's Decision Making Process*. Sudbury: HSE. Also available on the internet.

Jones-Lee M (1984) The valuation of transport safety, in *Proceedings of the Annual Transportation Convention*. Pretoria: Department of Transport.

Miller TR (1990) The plausible range for the value of life – red herrings among the mackerel. *Journal of Forensic Economics* 3(3): 17–39.

Soby B and Ball DJ (1991) *Consumer Safety and the Valuation of Life and Injury*. Research report No. 9. University of East Anglia Environmental Risk Assessment Unit. Brighton: UEA.

Stevens G, Wilson A and Hammitt JK (2005) A benefit-cost analysis of retrofitting diesel vehicles with particulate filters in the Mexico City Metropolitan Area. *Risk Analysis* 25(4): 883–99.

Turner RK, Pearce D and Bateman I (1994) *Environmental Economics: An Elementary Introduction*. Hemel Hempstead: Harvester Wheatsheaf.

9 The management of ionizing radiation

Overview

In several respects, ionizing radiation is important for anyone seeking an understanding of environmental health policy. First, it presents a hazard which, because it is naturally occurring as well as anthropogenic, affects everyone wherever they live. Second, much work and thought has gone into devising a framework which can be used for decision making about exposures to ionizing radiation and an understanding of this is extremely helpful. Third, the framework has been developed internationally through the work of agencies such as the International Commission on Radiological Protection (ICRP), the United Nations Scientific Committee on the Effects of Atomic Radiation (UNSCEAR) and the International Atomic Energy Agency (IAEA), and thus has global influence.

In this chapter you will see how this framework is assembled, including how it incorporates and builds upon the previous chapter on economic appraisal.

Learning objectives

By the end of this chapter, you will be better able to:

* **describe the sources and consequences of exposure to ionizing radiation**
* **distinguish between the various units by which radiation doses are measured**
* **discuss the associated framework for public health policy decision making**
* **understand the thinking behind and importance of the concepts of dose limits and optimization.**

Key terms

α value The monetary value of the man-sievert.

As low as reasonably achievable (ALARA) A fundamental concept in radiological protection, sometimes known as 'optimization'.

Collective dose The sum of the radiation doses to the individuals within a specified group, measured in units called man-sieverts.

Deterministic effects Effects which can be directly associated with their causes and which generally increase as dose increases. Normally a threshold exists.

Dose equivalent A measure of the amount of radiation absorbed by tissue combined with a factor accounting for the ability of the type of radiation involved to cause damage, measured in units called sieverts.

Dose limit The officially recognized maximum tolerable dose of ionizing radiation during a specified time interval.

Effective dose equivalent The dose equivalent incorporating a further weighting to account for the vulnerability to harm of the body part exposed, measured in units called sieverts.

Ionizing radiation Radiation that is sufficiently energetic to break the bonds that hold molecules together to form ions.

Sievert (Sv) A unit of equivalent dose of radiation which relates the absorbed dose in human tissue to the effective biological damage of the radiation. A millisievert (mSv) is one-thousandth of a sievert.

Stochastic effects Effects that are governed by the laws of probability. The severity of harm is independent of dose, but the probability of experiencing the harm is proportional to the dose. There is no threshold dose below which effects do not occur.

The nature of ionizing radiation

Some knowledge of the nature, origin and effects of ionizing radiation is required to get the most out of this chapter and the following three passages give a brief overview.

Radioactivity is a natural part of the universe in which we live and life on Earth would not exist without it. Nonetheless, it can be harmful, particularly at high doses, and its association with health effects like cancer and human activities like the manufacture of nuclear weapons has contributed to a widespread societal concern. It is likely this concern, coupled with the scientific and philosophical backgrounds of the people who have worked to understand ionizing radiation, has led to the evolution of the framework for assessing and managing the associated risks.

Ionizing radiation originates from atoms and their nuclei. For our purposes, atoms may be considered as made up of negatively-charged particles called electrons which orbit a small central nucleus which is made up of positively-charged protons and neutrons which have no charge (Figure 9.1). Each substance or element is characterized by the number of protons in the nucleus. For example, hydrogen has just one proton in its nucleus (it also has no neutrons and one orbiting electron. In its normal state the number of electrons equals the number of protons so that the charge on the total atom is zero.) In the case of uranium, this has 92 protons (and an equal number of orbiting electrons in its normal uncharged state). However, each element, hydrogen, uranium, oxygen, carbon or whatever, while being defined by the number of protons on the nucleus, may have different numbers of neutrons. So, for example, uranium comes in two well-known forms which are uranium-238 and uranium-235, known as isotopes of uranium. Uranium-238 is so called because it has 92 protons and 146 neutrons in its nucleus, while uranium–235 has 92 protons and 143 neutrons. These atoms, described in this way, are called 'nuclides'.

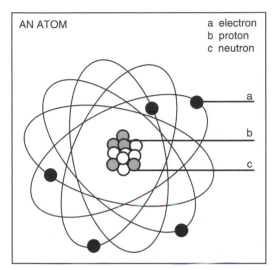

Figure 9.1 The atomic structure
Source: UNEP (1985)

Some nuclides of some elements are stable and never change, but most are not. They lose chunks in the form of protons, neutrons, electrons, or pure energy in the form of electromagnetic radiation, and are said to 'decay'. Simply speaking, there are three types of decay or emissions to consider, and these are known as alpha, beta and gamma (α, β, γ). *Alpha particles* are made up of a group of two protons and two neutrons, *beta particles* are electrons, and gamma emissions, known as *gamma rays*, are pure energy in the form of high energy electromagnetic radiation (like X-rays, but of higher energy). Figure 9.2 shows these emissions and also draws attention to the fact that they have very different penetrating power. Thus α particles cannot even penetrate a sheet of paper, nor even the top layer of human skin, so they are not dangerous to health unless the sources get inside the body through being inhaled or eaten as a part of the diet. β particles are more penetrating and can

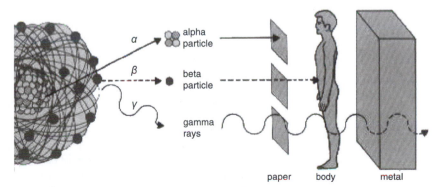

Figure 9.2 The three types of atomic radiation and their penetrating power
Source: UNEP (1985)

pass through a centimetre of living tissue, and γ rays can go through anything short of a thick slab of lead or concrete.

Activity 9.1

Damage to living tissue is caused by the energy deposited by the radiation as it passes through and disrupts human cells and damages DNA, and this is called the 'dose'. Dose is, however, a complicated concept in radiological protection. Read the following passage based on the United Nations Environment Programme (1985) description, and observe the different ways in which it is expressed.

Radiation measurement units

The amount of radiation energy that is absorbed per gram of tissue is called the absorbed dose and is measured in units called Grays (Gy). But this does not tell the full story because the same dose of α radiation is much more damaging than one of β or γ radiation. So the dose needs to be weighted for its potential to do damage, with α radiation given twenty times the weight of the others. This weighted dose is known as the 'dose equivalent' and is measured in units called sieverts (sv) (see Table 9.1 for a summary of the measurement units).

There is another refinement to be made. Some parts of the body are more vulnerable than others; a given dose of radiation is more likely to cause fatal cancer in the lung than in the thyroid, for example, and the reproductive organs are of particular concern because of the risk of genetic damage. The different parts of the body are therefore also given different weightings. Once it has been weighted appropriately, the 'dose equivalent' becomes the 'effective dose equivalent', also measured in sieverts.

This, however, describes only individual doses. If you add up all the individual effective dose equivalents received by a group of people, the result is called 'the collective effective dose equivalent' and this is expressed in man-sieverts (man-sv). But one further definition must be introduced because many radionuclides decay so slowly that they are radioactive far into the future. This is the collective effective dose equivalent that will be delivered to generations of people over time, and it is called 'the collective effective dose equivalent commitment'.

Table 9.1 Commonly-used units of measurement

Unit	Definition
Becquerel (Bq)	This is the name for the unit of activity of a radioactive material. The activity is the total number of α, β, or γ emissions per second. One becquerel corresponds to one disintegration per second of any radionuclide.
Gray (Gy)	The name for the unit of absorbed dose. It is the quantity of energy imparted by ionizing radiation to a unit mass of matter such as human tissue. One gray corresponds to one joule per kilogram.
Sievert (sv)	The name of a unit of dose equivalent. This is the absorbed dose weighted according to the potential of the radiation involved (α, β or γ) to do damage. One sievert also corresponds to one joule per kilogram.

Feedback

Doses are expressed in different ways to take account of how much of the body and what parts of it are irradiated, whether one or more people are exposed, and the duration of the exposure. The hierarchy is a little complicated but once understood it can be seen to provide a coherent structure against which doses can be recorded consistently and comparably.

The human effects and sources of radiation exposure

Radiation is harmful to life even at low doses because it can start off a chain of events which can lead to cancer or genetic damage (Figure 9.3), effects which may not reveal themselves until decades later. At high doses it can kill cells and damage organs, causing death within a few hours or days.

The acute effects of high doses occur after exposure above a certain threshold which is in the region of 1 Gray. Environmental exposures, from natural or man-made sources, are generally very much lower than this, by a factor of 1,000 or so. But in theory at least even the smallest dose poses an increased risk of cancer and genetic harm because ionizing radiation is taken to be a non-threshold agent.

Exposure can occur in two basic ways. First, people can be irradiated by external

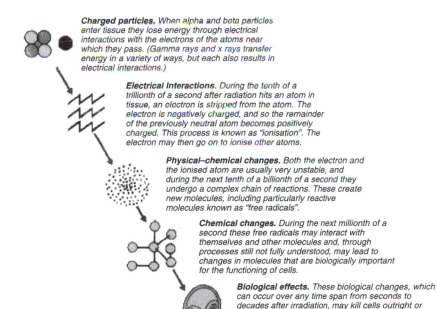

Charged particles. When alpha and beta particles enter tissue they lose energy through electrical interactions with the electrons of the atoms near which they pass. (Gamma rays and x rays transfer energy in a variety of ways, but each also results in electrical interactions.)

Electrical Interactions. During the tenth of a trillionth of a second after radiation hits an atom in tissue, an electron is stripped from the atom. The electron is negatively charged, and so the remainder of the previously neutral atom becomes positively charged. This process is known as "ionisation". The electron may then go on to ionise other atoms.

Physical–chemical changes. Both the electron and the ionised atom are usually very unstable, and during the next tenth of a billionth of a second they undergo a complex chain of reactions. These create new molecules, including particularly reactive molecules known as "free radicals".

Chemical changes. During the next millionth of a second these free radicals may interact with themselves and other molecules and, through processes still not fully understood, may lead to changes in molecules that are biologically important for the functioning of cells.

Biological effects. These biological changes, which can occur over any time span from seconds to decades after irradiation, may kill cells outright or alter them in ways that may lead to cancer and genetic effects.

Figure 9.3 How radiation affects tissue

Source: UNEP (1985)

sources. Second, people may be irradiated internally if they ingest or inhale dust, food, or water which contains trace amounts of radioactive materials.

By far the greatest contribution to the radiation exposure of the world's population is from natural sources. These sources are mainly of terrestrial origin, with the remaining roughly 10 per cent coming from outer space in the form of cosmic rays. The Earth's atmosphere shields us from most of the cosmic rays, but exposure increases for people living at high altitude or who fly frequently. For people living at sea level, the effective dose equivalent is about 0.3 millisieverts (one millisievert is $\frac{1}{1000}$ sievert) of cosmic radiation per year.

Of the terrestrial sources, radionuclides naturally present in rocks give rise to an average annual dose of about 0.35 millisieverts. There is some variation across the planet, due to the make-up of the rocks, and 'hotspots' have been found at places like Poços de Caldas in Brazil (250 millisieverts per year and thankfully uninhabited) and parts of Kerala and Tamil Nadu in India (up to 17 millisieverts per year).

The above sources are all external and together contribute about one-quarter of total exposure. The other three-quarters are down to internal irradiation which results from naturally occurring radioactive substances in food, air and water. These include potassium-40, lead-210 and polonium-210 which enter the body in food. Although the average dose per person worldwide from such sources is about 0.3 millisieverts, some of these materials are concentrated in certain foodstuffs like seafood, and kangaroo and caribou meat where these animals graze in areas naturally rich in them, so local populations can receive higher doses. However, the largest natural source of radiation exposure worldwide is the gas radon which exists as a minor constituent of the atmosphere. Radon primarily originates from the radioactive decay of naturally occurring uranium-238 in the ground and seeps from the earth into the air. The concentration in the air depends on the amount of uranium-238 in the ground, and it can be higher inside well-insulated, draught-proofed buildings where it sometimes accumulates. Exposure therefore depends on the kind of buildings in which people live and the ground on which they are built. It is not so much the radon itself which is the problem, but that it undergoes quite rapid radioactive decay into polonium-218 and polonium-214 which, if the radon gas has been inhaled, can lodge in the lung and are α-emitters. The emission of α particles in such a sensitive area of the body increases the risk of lung cancer. Doses attributable to radon decay are typically about 1.3 millisieverts per year, but can be hundreds or thousands of times higher in special circumstances.

Doses from man-made radiation are usually much smaller than from natural radiation, but vary considerably. In countries that practise Western-style medicine, the largest source of exposure to the public is the use of X-rays and radioactive materials to diagnose and combat disease, and average doses to the public of around 0.3 millisieverts in a year from this source are normal. Occupational exposure, through working in hospitals or industry, is highly regulated and exposures are typically in the range from 0.1 to 0.3 millisieverts per year. The nuclear and other industries, hospitals and universities discharge some radioactivity to the atmosphere in routine operation, but the resulting public exposures are generally low and below 0.001 millisieverts per year. One other source which should be mentioned is nuclear fallout from previous but now ceased atmospheric testing of nuclear weapons. Doses to the public were typically around 0.14

millisieverts per annum in the early 1960s but have by now fallen to less than 0.005 millisieverts. Figure 9.4 shows the average relative importance of the various natural and man-made sources as pertaining for the UK population. Table 9.2 shows worldwide average annual effective doses.

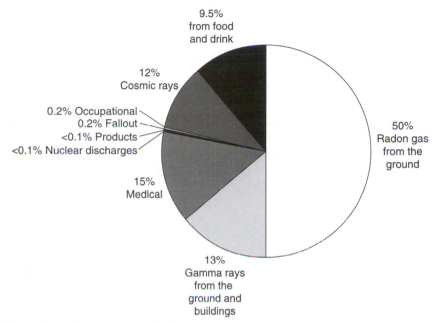

Figure 9.4 The main sources of radiation exposure in the United Kingdom

Source: HPA Centre (2006)

Table 9.2 Average radiation doses at year 2000 from natural and man-made sources of radiation expressed in millisieverts (msv) per annum

Source	Worldwide average annual effective dose (msv/annum)
Natural background	2.4
Diagnostic medical examinations	0.4
Atmospheric nuclear testing	0.005
Chernobyl accident	0.002
Nuclear power production	0.002

Source: UNSCEAR (2000)

The health implications of radiation exposure

In the time since the health aspects of radiation have been a topic of research a great deal of work has been conducted to try and identify the risks. A primary interest has been the shape of the dose–response curve at low doses. The main source of information has been the lifespan study of the survivors of Hiroshima and Nagasaki which was most recently reported and assessed by UNSCEAR in 2000. As a result of this and other research, UNSCEAR estimates that the risk of dying from cancer at low or moderate doses is in the range of 4–6 per cent per sievert of radiation exposure. Research on the health effects of radiation is a continuing business and it is possible that this risk factor could change in the light of new information.

 Activity 9.2

Using information from the above passages:

1 What would be the additional lifetime risk of contracting fatal cancer for a hypothetical person who lived at Poços de Caldas for one year?
2 What is the collective dose of the UK population of 60 million from radon exposure and how many cases of fatal cancer would be expected annually from this hazard?
3 Identify an important assumption in making these estimates.

 Feedback

1 The dose resulting from one year's exposure at Poços de Caldas would be 250 msv. Using UNSCEAR's risk factor of 4–6 per cent risk per sievert of exposure, the additional lifetime risk would be given by:

$$\text{from } (250 \times 10^{-3}) \times 4/100 \text{ to } (250 \times 10^{-3}) \times 6/100$$
$$\text{or from } 0.01 \text{ to } 0.015 \text{ (i.e. from } 1–1.5\%)$$

2 Taking the annual individual dose from radon to be 1.3 msv, the collective dose is given by:

$$(1.3 \times 10^{-3}) \times (60 \times 10^{6}) = 78{,}000 \text{ man-sv}$$

and the expected annual number of cases would be:

$$\text{from } (78{,}000 \times 4/100) \text{ to } (78{,}000 \times 6/100)$$
$$\text{or from about } 3{,}000 \text{ to } 5{,}000$$

3 These estimates, particularly for the UK example, are dealing with low doses and are dependent on the validity of the LNT hypothesis discussed in Chapter 5. It is of interest to note that if the calculations in 2 are correct, then as many people in the UK die from exposure to background levels of radon as are killed in road traffic accidents or in the workplace.

The principles of radiation protection

The aim of radiation protection is to provide a good standard of safety for people exposed to ionizing radiation but without limiting its beneficial uses or disrupting everyday life. In 1977, the ICRP issued the following recommendations for this purpose:

- no practice shall be adopted unless its introduction produces a positive net benefit;
- all exposures shall be kept *as low as reasonably achievable* (ALARA), economic and social factors being taken into account;
- the dose equivalent to individuals shall not exceed the limits recommended for the appropriate circumstances by the Commission.

These three principles are commonly referred to as justification, optimization and limitation. An understanding of them is important for public health policy makers, even those not working in radiological protection, because of the ideas that underpin them and that have much wider purpose. The main interest from the health policy perspective is in the second and third principles which will now be examined.

Optimization and the meaning of the ALARA principle

In many aspects of life, particularly those turning points where big decisions have to be made, you will encounter the need to weigh up the advantages or disadvantages of any particular course of action before deciding what to do. In some professional circles the formal term for this procedure is 'optimization'. You have already come across it in Chapter 8 of this book, because cost–benefit analysis is one method of optimizing decisions. In radiation protection, ALARA, the ICRP concept that all radiation doses shall be kept As Low As Reasonably Achievable, economic and social factors being taken into account, is consistent with choosing the best course of action in given circumstances. Thus, in radiation protection:

ALARA = optimization of radiation protection

 Activity 9.3

The following extract from Stokell et al. (1991) discusses the ALARA concept and its origins. As you read it, consider:

1 Why did radiation protection switch from a system based purely upon exposure limits to one incorporating optimization (ALARA)?
2 What were the driving forces behind the development of the ALARA principle?
3 What is the difference between deterministic effects and stochastic (probabilistic) effects? Give an example of each.
4 Is the aim of radiation protection dose minimization?

 Optimisation of radiation protection

In the early days of radiation protection it was believed that if an individual's radiation dose were kept below a certain threshold level, then there was no hazard to his health. This belief originated in the observation of non-stochastic or deterministic effects, where people exposed to sufficiently large doses of radiation, either X-rays or from radioactive material, incurred damage to tissue, but that at low doses no effects were observed. Based on this, early systems of radiation protection were directed at keeping an individual's dose below dose limits that were defined with reference to the threshold for these effects.

In time it was realised that there were other health consequences from radiation exposure, both somatic (in the exposed individual himself) and genetic (in his offspring), that appeared to show no observable threshold dose. These effects are termed stochastic or probabilistic, and it was assumed that an increased radiation dose implied an increased likelihood of suffering one of these effects. It was also assumed that this relationship held down to zero dose, i.e. even at very low levels of dose there remained a possibility, however small, of sustaining one of these health effects . . .

Acknowledging that there was no completely 'safe' level of radiation exposure led to the idea that the best one could do would be to reduce radiation exposures as far as possible. However, radiation protection, like many other practices, is subject to the law of diminishing returns – an initial expenditure on protection may result in a significant dose reduction, but further expenditure produces progressively smaller reductions. Since there are never infinite resources available to spend on protection, the question arises as to how far one should go in reducing doses. Control has to be achieved on the basis of some sort of trade-off between the reduction in radiation exposure and the cost of the protective measures that could be taken. In other words, there is a need for some sort of optimisation of radiation protection.

 Feedback

1 The switch was made when it was discovered that for some effects, cancer and hereditary consequences, radiation was a non-threshold agent.

2 The development of the ALARA principle is driven by two factors. These are the absence of a threshold dose and the fact that resources for radiation protection are not unlimited.

3 Living or working in a dusty environment which exceeds a certain threshold concentration will inevitably lead to a reduction in lung function, and this reduction is likely to increase as dose increases. Such would be a deterministic relationship. Asbestos workers may in this way suffer asbestosis and smokers may contract emphysema. In contrast, both asbestos workers and smokers *might* contract cancer, though this is not certain and can only be stated in terms of probabilities. Stochastic effects have no threshold.

4 Radiation protection is *not* about dose minimization. It is about striking a balance between dose limitation and resource allocation.

It is worth noting that although the concept of ALARA stems from the absence of a demonstrable threshold for stochastic effects, that even if a threshold were shown to exist, a trade-off between the benefits of dose reduction and costs of achieving those reductions would still be required at levels above that threshold (Figure 9.5).

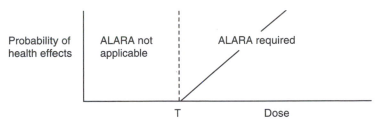

Figure 9.5 Even if there were a threshold (T) in the dose–response curve, the ALARA principle would still apply at doses above the threshold

Source: Stokell et al. (1991)

Deciding what is 'reasonably achievable'

The ICRP's second principle requires you to decide how much effort should reasonably be invested in reducing radiation exposure.

 Activity 9.4

From what you already know, can you outline a method for determining quantitatively the levels of radiation protection which could be described as reasonably achievable in any given circumstance?

 Feedback

To answer this, look back at Chapter 8. If it were possible to put a monetary value on the impairment to health resulting from radiation exposure (as was done for the value of a life), the value of the health benefits of any exposure reductions could be calculated, and these could then be compared with the costs of interventions used to bring them about. Interventions satisfying the ALARA principle could then be identified as those giving rise to potential Pareto improvements.

 Activity 9.5

Read the following extract based upon David Ball and Geoffrey Goats (1996) which describes the approach in the UK to valuing the harmful effects of radiation exposures and make notes of how it links up with Chapter 8.

 Valuing the effects of radiation exposure

During the period 1985 to 1989 the National Radiological Protection Board (NRPB) recommended a base-line value of £3,000 per man-Sv. The value of the man-sievert is sometimes referred to as the α (alpha) value. This sum reflected the pecuniary costs of lost output, health care and other matters associated with the stochastic effects in irradiated populations. The Board also recommended that its minimum base-line cost of a unit collective dose be multiplied by an additional factor, either equal to or greater than

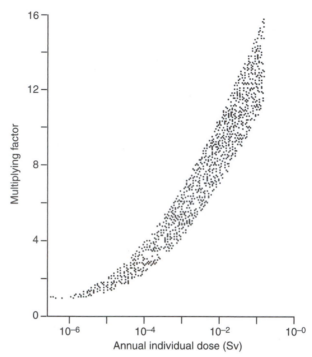

Figure 9.6 The NRPB's risk aversion factor
Note: The curve is 'fuzzy' because of recognized uncertainties.
Source: NRPB (1993)

unity, related to the individual dose distributions encountered in specific circumstances. The factor was intended to reflect only the aspect of individual risk aversion towards increasing levels of individual dose. Figure 9.6 shows the recommended value for the multiplication factor ... within the range of effective dose equivalents from 10^{-6} to about 1 sv.

In 1993 an important change was incorporated into the calculation of the base-line value of a unit of collective dose (i.e. the cost per man-sievert or the α value) for premature death or ill-health, and of genetic damage. This was because the 'human capital' approach, upon which the value of £3,000 per man-sievert had been based, had received some criticism. This occurred because the fundamental premise of the theory of welfare economics is that public sector allocative decisions should reflect as far as possible the informed preferences of those who will be affected by the decision, in other words, their willingness to pay (WTP).

The Board took note of the fact that 'values of life' emerging from WTP-based studies were higher than those based on human capital and that a median value was about £1.6 million. On the assumption that the average age of all the study populations was 38 years, it could be supposed that the remaining life expectancy was 39 years. Thus, the value of a life-year (VOLY) would be £1.6 million/39, or approximately £40,000. Bearing in mind the uncertainty, the NRPB adopted a range for the VOLY of £40,000 to £60,000 (without discounting).

Using the latest data on radiation-induced health risks, an average weighted years of life lost (YOLL) per unit collective dose was calculated for the population of England and

Wales. The value of YOLL was found to be about 1.0 years per sievert. Thus, the implied value of the man-sievert at the risk level of the WTP studies is about £30,000 to £60,000.

To calculate a base-line value of α, it was necessary to bear in mind that the WTP studies were carried out on populations facing an average risk of about 1×10^{-4} per annum. In radiation terms this would be equivalent to a dose of a few mSv which, from Figure 9.6, is associated with a risk aversion multiplier of about 5 to 7. Thus, the base-line value of the man-Sievert which would apply at very low dose levels where the aversion multiplier was close to unity would be in the range of £5,000 to £12,000.

 Feedback

The NRPB's approach is clearly consistent with using a welfare economics-based model for health policy decision making. Such an approach would benefit from having recognized monetary valuations of health detriments which result from the typical, low-level, exposures that people receive, either in the environment or at work. Thus, they sought to value the basic unit of radiation exposure, the man-sievert. First, NRPB used the human capital (lost earnings) approach for valuing the man-sievert, but switched to WTP when that went out of fashion. The Board did not have its own WTP survey data and instead took a median value for a life from other WTP studies of non-radiological risks. This was then crudely converted, without discounting, to a value of a life-year, so it was then fairly straightforward to put a price on a man-sievert by using an estimate of the average number of life-years lost per man-sievert of exposure. One obvious complication is the use of the 'risk aversion' curve in Figure 9.6. NRPB felt that people are more averse to risk, the higher the level of risk they are exposed to. They speculated that the degree of risk aversion was as shown in Figure 9.6. They then considered that most people who had answered the original WTP questions would have been influenced by their personal level of risk from all sources. Typically this is taken to be about 1 in 10,000 risk of dying per year. They then deduced that this level of risk (using UNSCEAR's 4–6 per cent risk factor) was equivalent to a radiation exposure of about 2 millisv (msv), and from Figure 9.6 this can be seen to be equivalent to a risk aversion factor of 5–7. NRPB were interested in the valuation of α at much lower doses than this (with an aversion factor of unity) so that a 'baseline' value could be calculated. This would provide the minimum value of α, from which all other values, relevant at higher doses, could be calculated as required using Figure 9.6. The baseline value of α was calculated by dividing the value of α at 2 msv (£30,000 to £60,000) by this factor of 5 to 7.

While the details of the above calculation are somewhat complicated, the key point to note is that the ALARA approach is often closely connected with the use of CBA which in turn is based in the theory of welfare economics. Also be aware that the valuation of the man-sievert will, in addition to its dependence on dose, change with time as GNP (gross national product) changes, may vary from place to place depending on local GNP and other social factors, and also if methodologies or risk factors change. Figure 9.7 shows the results of a survey of α values as used in different countries in 2002 (ISOE 2003), all expressed in Euros per man-millisievert (equivalent to α/1,000).

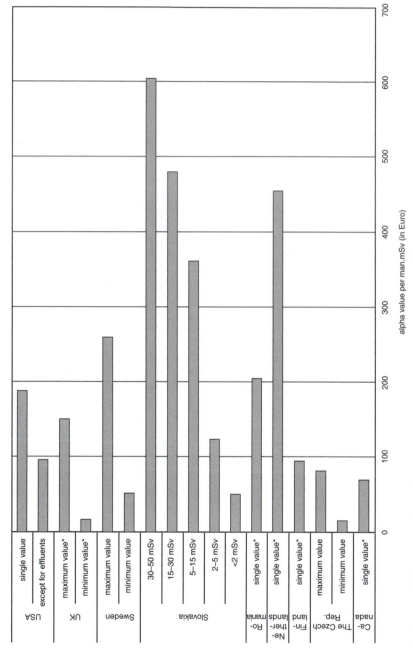

Figure 9.7 Alpha values adopted by regulatory agencies in different countries (*1997 survey)

Source: ISOE (2003)

Dose limits

The third principle of the ICRP is concerned with 'dose limits'. The aim of dose limits is to set levels of exposure to ionizing radiation which should not be exceeded for any individual.

 Activity 9.6

Reflect upon why it is necessary to set dose limits when radiation exposures are already constrained by the ALARA principle.

 Feedback

ALARA is concerned with maximizing the overall welfare of a group of people. As with Kaldor and Hicks' modification of the Pareto principle, it is about *potential* Pareto improvements. In these circumstances a change may make some individuals worse off than others, yet still be seen as a good thing because the collective welfare of the group is increased. The concept of dose limits is therefore introduced as a safety net to ensure that no individual experiences risks which would, on ethical grounds, be deemed unacceptable by society.

The setting of dose limits is only partially a scientific task because it relies upon judgements. A widely used value for the dose limit for members of the public is 1 millisievert per year. This usually applies to all controlled sources, but not natural radiation which, at a global average of 2.4 millisieverts per annum, is clearly higher. For workers, a dose limit value of 20 millisieverts per year is commonly used. Where do these values come from? Using the mid-point (5 per cent) of the UNSCEAR risk factor of 4–6 per cent per sievert, it can be seen that the dose limit for workers is equivalent to an annual risk of dying (from fatal cancer) of about:

$$(20 \times 10^{-3}) \times 5\% = 1/1000$$

Occupational risks of dying of 1 in 1000 per annum are fairly widely regarded as the maximum risks that workers should be exposed to. Studies of the risks that workers face in dangerous jobs, like mining, quarrying or deep sea fishing, generally show that the levels of risk experienced are of this order and it is considered that this is the maximum tolerable risk which workers should have to face. This then is the justification for the dose limit of 20 mSv per annum for workers. It should be noted that this by no means implies that workers can therefore be exposed to what some people would regard as a high level of risk without further thought. This is because the second principle, that all exposures shall be kept as low as reasonably achievable (ALARA), economic and social factors being taken into account, is there to continually drive down any risk to lower levels.

In the case of the public, the dose limit of 1 millisievert per annum is 20 times lower than that for workers. The justification given for this is that the public is involuntarily exposed to these risks, whereas workers are paid and are aware of the risk.

Second, workers are generally fitter and healthier than the wider population and may be more resilient.

An overview

Figure 9.8 sets out the components of the underlying philosophy of radiological protection. It is possible to think of radiation dose, and its associated risk, as falling into one of three domains. In Figure 9.8, the top domain of highest dose is deemed to pose an unacceptable risk under any normal circumstances, and this region is defined by dose limits. The central domain is one where risk is sufficiently high to be of concern, but may be tolerated in exchange for benefits of activities or because the cost and difficulty of control are too much. Where the correct balance of control lies is determined by application of the ALARA principle. Risks (doses) *must* be reduced until as low as reasonably achievable. There is also potentially a third domain of very low doses which are not of concern to people because the risks are so small. You will read more about this in Chapter 10.

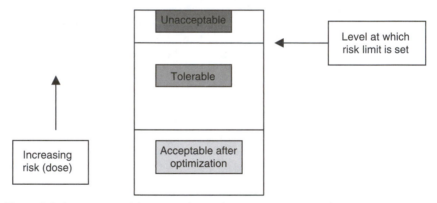

Figure 9.8 An overview of the approach to radiation exposure control

Summary

This chapter has introduced a basic framework against which decisions about radiological protection can be made, taking account of the benefits of reducing exposures to risk and the opportunity cost of doing this. The framework has two essential ingredients: dose limits and ALARA. The concept of dose limits, or maximum tolerable risk, is there to protect all individuals from unreasonable exposure to risk of harm. The second ingredient, ALARA, is an acronym for 'all doses shall be kept as low as reasonably achievable, economic and social factors being taken into account'. In radiation protection circles, it is synonymous with 'optimization'. The ALARA principle is a direct consequence of the absence of a threshold for health effects and the fact that resources are limited. Often decisions in radiation protection can be made without recourse to complex calculation and are based on experience, but a logical framework is always helpful in achieving uniformity. In this chapter, cost–benefit analysis was used as a tool for identifying optimal control, but other techniques are available and will be introduced later. The ALARA procedure is merely an aid to decision making and the final choice still remains the responsibility of the decision maker.

References

Ball DJ and Goats G (1996). Risk management and consumer safety. International Journal for Consumer Safety 3(3): 111–24.

Health Protection Agency Centre for Radiation, Chemical and Environmental Hazards (2005).

ICRP (1977) Recommendations of the International Commission on Radiological Protection, ICRP Publication 26. *Ann. ICRP* 1(3). Oxford: Pergamon Press.

ISOE European Technical Centre (2003) *Man-Sievert Monetary Value Survey (2002 update)*. Information sheet No. 34. Paris: CEPN.

Stokell PJ, Croft JR, Lochard J and Lombard J (1991) *Radiation protection: ALARA from Theory to Practice*. Luxembourg: Office for Official Publications of the Commission of the European Communities.

UNEP (1985) *Radiation: Doses, Effects, Risks*. Nairobi: UNEP.

UNSCEAR (2000) *Sources and Effects of Ionizing Radiation*. New York: Report to the UN General Assembly.

10 | Environment and safety

Overview

In the previous chapter you were introduced to a framework for making health policy decisions about ionizing radiation. The framework was found to be based on risk (or dose) limits, and exposure control through the process of managing risks according to the principle of ALARA. In this chapter you will look at two other areas of health policy: public and occupational safety from risk of injury, and environmental health. The aim is to see if parallel approaches exist, and if so, the extent to which there is a general framework for making environmental health policy decisions.

Learning objectives

By the end of this chapter, you will be better able to:

- **outline approaches to occupational and public safety and environmental health**
- **understand the concepts of *de minimis* and *de manifestis* risk and their significance**
- **describe an overall framework of environmental health policy formulation.**

Key terms

As low as reasonably practicable (ALARP) In some countries a fundamental concept in safety assessment.

Best available technique not entailing excessive cost (BATNEEC) A pollution control philosophy.

Best practicable environmental option (BPEO) A pollution control philosophy.

de manifestis When applied to risk, refers to levels that are manifestly intolerable.

de minimis When applied to risk, refers to levels that are considered trivial or negligible.

Public and occupational safety and injury prevention

Injury prevention might appear to be an unusual place to pick up the story of environmental health policy, but it is an area which, in recent years, has seen a surge of interest. In practice, injuries rank among the leading causes of death and burden of disease and occur in all regions and countries, affecting people of all ages and income groups (WHO 2002). The hazards giving rise to injuries vary with age, gender, income and region. For example, in the low- and middle-income regions of the western Pacific, the leading injury-related causes of death are road traffic accidents and interpersonal violence, while in the low- and middle-income countries of Europe suicide and poisoning are more important.

An interesting question is perhaps why until now injuries have not received greater attention in the public health sector, to which Judith Green (1997) provides a fascinating response from a sociological perspective. The simple answer, though, is that injuries have traditionally been regarded as random, unavoidable events – accidents in the usual sense of the word – thus having little prospect of being either understood or prevented. However, the epidemiology of accidents is now well established and this shows that accidents appear not as unique misfortunes, but as statistically predictable events with identifiable social, environmental, psychological and biological risk factors (Green 1997). As a result of this shift in perception, injuries and their health implications have increasingly attracted the attention of decision makers worldwide and injury policy has found its place on the public health agenda. The World Health Organization, for example, has established a Department of Injury and Violence prevention.

 Activity 10.1

While reading the following passage from the World Health Organization (2002), consider who should be involved in injury prevention programmes and what factors should be taken into account in policy formulation.

When you have finished reading, make some notes in response to the following questions:

1 Why do you think that WHO recommends involving non-government persons in injury prevention?
2 Are prioritization and resource allocation recognized as important issues?
3 What factors might account for the uneven development of injury prevention strategies around the world?

 National injury prevention policies

Several governments around the world have developed national injury prevention policies, strategies and/or plans of action. Although these instruments vary in nature and scope, they serve to guide a nation's efforts to prevent injury-related death and disability. WHO's *World report on road traffic injury prevention* and *World report on violence and health* call upon Member States to develop such tools for the prevention of road traffic injuries and violence respectively. WHO recommends that such policies, strategies and plans of action be concrete and contain objectives, priorities, timetables and mechanisms for evaluation. WHO suggests that responsibility be assigned for all stages of their implementation and that they be developed in a participatory manner, involving both government and non-government actors alike. Some policies are developed by and for a single sector such as health, transport, justice or education, but ideally they should be developed in a multi-sectoral fashion. It is also recommended that policy makers and planners take into account at an early stage the human and financial requirements that will be necessary for their implementation.

Most national injury prevention policies, strategies and/or plans of action currently in use around the world originate in high-income countries. Few low- and middle-income countries have such policies, although more have been developed in recent years. Of those which presently exist, some are comprehensive pertaining to all injury-related mortality and morbidity, while others focus on a particular type of injury such as road traffic injuries or violence-related injuries or a particular group of intended beneficiaries such as children, youth or women. Much depends on the burden posed by these public health concerns in the country and the country's willingness and ability to recognize these as issues which need to be addressed and to take action.

 Feedback

1 Involving non-governmental parties is a modern trend in some societies and one which we will consider more carefully in Chapter 17. There are three basic reasons for it: (1) useful practical things might be learned by involving people outside of government; (2) it is in the interests of democracy to involve people in policy making; and (3) if people are invited to help in policy making, then they are more likely to accept the policy, and support it, when it comes to implementation.

2 Once again, it can be seen that resource allocation, human or financial, is recognized as an appropriate issue by the WHO, as it is by other national and international agencies. Policy decisions, even about things as important as health and safety, cannot avoid being scrutinized and prioritized.

3 There are many factors which might account for uneven development of injury prevention strategies. They range from societal beliefs about the nature of accidents and their preventability, to the agendas of professions and health protection agencies, and the level of organization, type of infrastructure, and resources. Injury prevention has only in the past few decades been recognized as a legitimate field of activity, and it is therefore not surprising if some areas have yet to pick up the banner. Of course, they might also have other more pressing concerns.

A framework for injury prevention policy

Increasingly the accepted approach to injury control is regarded as being through the identification of hazards and the assessment of the level of risks and consequences associated with each hazard (using definitions of hazard and risk as given in Chapter 3). The results are often displayed on a risk-consequence, or risk profile matrix as it is sometimes called, as shown in Figure 10.1 (note the similarity to Figure 7.1).

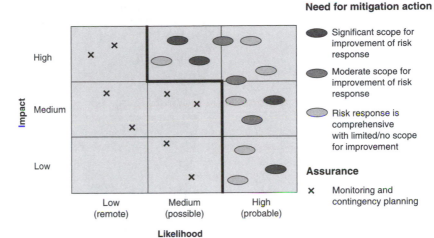

Figure 10.1 A typical risk profile matrix

Source: UK Cabinet Office (2002)

✏️ **Activity 10.2**

Figure 10.1 shows a number of interesting features. Each point drawn on the matrix corresponds to a specific hazard, e.g. a slippery or uneven floor, a broken electrical socket, a dangerous bend in a road, an unprotected drop, etc. The heavy line in Figure 10.1 can be compared with either the upper boundary of unacceptable risk or the lower boundary of acceptable risk in Figure 9.8. Which is it?

↻ **Feedback**

The line in question would have to correspond with the lower boundary of Figure 9.8 because if it were the upper boundary, the hazards above and to the right of the line would normally *require* action to move them to lower risk and consequence, but the implication in Figure 10.1 is that this is not necessarily the case, for example, if there is limited scope for improvement. It is as if an achievability criterion, as in ALARA, is being considered for the hazards shown.

The following edited passage from an article by David Ball and Geoffrey Goats (1996) describes a framework, shown in Figure 10.2, and sometimes referred to as the 'Tolerability of Risk (ToR) framework', against which occupational safety is assessed in the United Kingdom. This approach is also seen as relevant in decision making about risks to the public. The vertical axis in Figure 10.2 is the level of risk of death by injury, with high risk at the top.

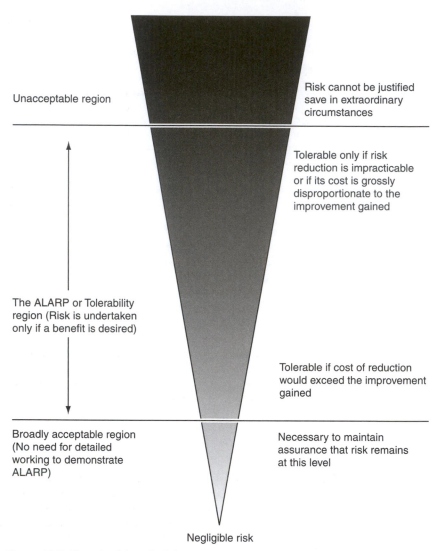

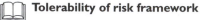

Negligible risk

Figure 10.2 The tolerability of risk framework

Note: In this diagram there is a reference to 'gross disproportion'. This is a British legal concept which is of limited relevance here and is therefore not discussed.

Source: HSE (1988)

Tolerability of risk framework

Figure 10.2 is helpful in comprehending the approach to risk control which is taken by the UK Health and Safety Executive (HSE), and in the guidance which it provides to risk managers. With reference to Figure 10.2 it can be seen that the risks associated with an activity are first assessed against three criteria:

- whether a given risk is so great or the outcome so unacceptable that it must be refused altogether (top zone);
- whether a risk is, or has been made, so small that no further precaution is necessary (bottom zone);
- if a risk falls in the intermediate zone, that it has been reduced to the lowest level practicable, bearing in mind the benefits arising from its acceptance and taking into account the costs and difficulty of any further reduction.

Inherent within the scheme are a number of fundamental concepts. First, the idea of zero risk has been rejected. Instead, the notion of tolerating risks in exchange for the benefits of risky activities is introduced. Second, above a certain level a risk is regarded as intolerable and cannot be justified under any ordinary circumstances. Third, below the intolerable risk level an activity may take place provided that the associated risks have been reduced by all available methods that are *reasonably practicable*, i.e. risks have been reduced until as low as reasonably practicable (ALARP).

In considering whether further safety improvements are necessary to comply with the ALARP criterion, formal cost–benefit techniques can be applied. This requires monetary values to be placed on risk reductions.

At very low risk levels, referred to in Figure 10.2 as the 'broadly acceptable region', it may not be worth allocating further resources provided there is confidence that these levels of risk can be maintained in practice.

Activity 10.3

What are the similarities and dissimilarities between this approach and that used in radiological protection?

Feedback

They are comparable in a number of ways. The ALARA principle appears here as ALARP. While there are some minor differences between these principles, they are not relevant here. The principles are similar in that they require a balance to be made between the benefits of an intervention, whether to reduce risk of injury or radiation exposure, and the cost and difficulty of implementing the measures. Thus, ALARP and ALARA are underpinned by techniques such as monetary evaluation of health states and cost–benefit analysis for their formal implementation. The HSE's framework also sets upper and lower risk limits, analogous to the dose limits used in radiological protection.

Risk limits

The risk limits relating to the upper and lower boundaries in Figure 10.2 come from similar sources and by similar reasoning to that used in radiological protection. Regarding the upper limit, the boundary between intolerable and just-tolerable risk, the HSE observed that, broadly, an individual risk of death of 1 in 1,000 per annum is about the most that is ordinarily accepted under modern conditions for workers in the UK and that it seemed reasonable to adopt this figure as the dividing line between what is just tolerable and what is intolerable (HSE 1988). For the public, a lower figure of 1 in 10,000 was proposed, largely because these risks are involuntary from the public perspective.

As in the case of radiological protection, it could be argued that these are very high risks to set as criteria for tolerability, but the point is that hazards must also comply with the ALARP criterion. For hazards in the middle zone of Figure 10.2, all measures that are reasonably practicable must be implemented, and this will continue to drive risks down, but not in a never-ending way that requires infinite resources.

So far as the level of individual risk which might be considered broadly acceptable in Figure 10.2 is concerned, the HSE proposed that this could be taken as 1 in a million per annum, for both workers and the public, since this would constitute only a very small addition to the normal risks of life and was not a level of risk which people ordinarily worried about or took action over. It is, for example, roughly equivalent to the annual risk of being killed by a lightning strike.

International applicability

You have already noted that the approach adopted for radiological hazard management is international in scope through the participation of so many countries in agencies like the UNSCEAR, ICRP and IAEA. The same can be said of the broad details of the approach just described towards safety from accidents. Consider, for example, the International Maritime Organization (IMO) and the SOLAS (Safety of Life at Sea) Convention. IMO and SOLAS make use of the technique of Formal Safety Assessment (FSA) to identify, by a rational and systematic process, practicable control measures for implementation that increase safety and reduce pollution risks on the oceans while giving good value for money to stakeholders. Figure 10.3 shows the FSA methodology as described by the UK Maritime and Coastguard Agency (2006), with its embedded use of cost–benefit analysis which, in radiological protection, is called 'optimization'.

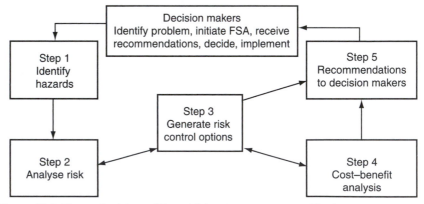

Figure 10.3 The methodology of Formal Safety Assessment as used by the IMO
Source: Maritime and Coastguard Agency (2006)

A framework for environmental health policy

You have now encountered health policy frameworks in the areas of radiological protection and injury prevention. Radiological hazards and hazards giving rise to injuries both fall within the general domain of public health, but there are many other areas too, including exposure to chemical and biological agents, natural or man-made, in the environment. The question is, do similar frameworks for risk management exist in these areas? The answer is, broadly, that they do. In fact, if you read the literature on environmental pollution control, you will come across terms such as BPEO (best practicable environmental option) and BATNEEC (best available technique not entailing excessive cost), both concepts having similarities to ALARA and ALARP.

The following edited extract from a document by David Kocher (1996) for the US Department of Energy proposes a general framework for risk management of both radionuclides and hazardous chemicals in the environment.

 Activity 10.4

As you read it, consider the following:

1 How do the concepts of *de minimis* and *de manifestis risk* fit in with the frameworks which have been described for radiological protection and injury prevention?
2 Can it be inferred that there is, at least in outline, a consistent philosophy with regard to health policy across the areas of radiological protection, hazardous environmental chemicals, and injury prevention?

 General framework for risk management

For any substances in the environment, current approaches to risk management generally recognize, either explicitly or implicitly, that risks to public health can be grouped into three broad categories. These categories are summarized in Table 10.1 and are described below.

The first of these categories, which is the subject discussed here, includes any risks that are considered *de minimis*. The term *de minimis* stems from the legal principle 'De minimis non curat lex', meaning 'The law does not concern itself with trifles.' Thus, as applied to radionuclides and hazardous chemicals in the environment, the term *de minimis*, refers to levels which are considered trivial or negligible, meaning that the associated risks to public health are so low that action to reduce risks generally is unwarranted.

The primary impetus for establishing *de minimis* levels of radionuclides and hazardous chemicals in the environment is the recognition that efforts at reducing risk generally are not cost-free. Rather, efforts at risk reduction for any exposure situation entail a direct monetary cost, and decisions thus are required about whether it is worth allocating resources to reduce risk. In addition, for remediation work, there may be other, more indirect costs including, for example, increased exposures of workers to the contaminants, damage to ecosystems and the environment, transfer of risks to other locations and populations, and a decrease in resources available for other beneficial purposes. The

Table 10.1 General framework for categorizing risks from exposure to radionuclides and hazardous chemicals in the environment

Severity of risk[a]	Characterization of risk	Approach to risk reduction
De minimis	Risks are so low that they are considered trivial or negligible.	Action to reduce risk generally is unwarranted.
Intermediate	Risks are between de minimis and de manifestis levels.	Feasibility of risk reduction generally must be considered, but action to reduce risk is required only if risks are above levels judged as low as reasonably achievable (ALARA).
De manifestis	Risks are so high that they are considered manifestly intolerable.	Action to reduce risk generally is required, regardless of cost or any other considerations.

Source: Kocher (1996)

Note: [a] Severity of risk increases from top to bottom of table.

concept of de minimis levels of hazardous substances in the environment then embodies the notion that, at sufficiently low levels of risk, it simply is not worth the cost of attempting to achieve further risk reduction, even if the required direct expenditures and other associated costs would not be large.

A second category, which is at the opposite end of the risk spectrum from de minimis levels, includes any risks that are considered de manifestis, which means that the risks are so high that they are manifestly intolerable. For risks in this category, action to reduce risk generally would be required under any circumstances (e.g. regardless of cost).

The third category includes any risks intermediate between de minimis and de manifestis. This category thus includes risks which are neither so low that they can be neglected nor so high that risk reduction would be required regardless of any other circumstances. For risks in this intermediate category, risk reduction generally must be considered because the risks are too high to be neglected out-of-hand, but risk reduction would be required only if it is feasible (e.g. cost-effective) because the risks are not so high that they are manifestly intolerable.

An important characteristic of risks in the intermediate category is that judgments are required on a case-by-case basis about the extent to which risks should be reduced. A general principle that is widely applied in controlling exposures to radionuclides and hazardous chemicals in the environment is that risks should be as low as reasonably achievable (ALARA), taking into account economic factors (i.e., cost–benefit) and other societal concerns. However, it must be emphasized that achieving a de minimis risk is not the goal of ALARA because risks that are ALARA may be well above de minimis levels. On the other hand, the ALARA principle generally would not be applied for risks at de minimis levels, even if risk reduction would be cost-effective, again because de minimis risks generally are too low to be of concern.

Particularly in current approaches to risk management for hazardous chemicals, risks at de minimis levels often are referred to as 'acceptable'. However, the three categories of risk described above and summarized in Table 10.1 serve to emphasize that risks above de minimis levels also can be acceptable under certain conditions – namely, if the risks are not so high that they are manifestly intolerable and they are ALARA. Thus, it is improper to characterize all risks above de minimis levels as 'unacceptable', because such risks are unacceptable only if they are manifestly intolerable or they are below manifestly intolerable levels but are not ALARA.

Feedback

1 The *de minimis* and *de manifestis* concepts fit neatly with the dose limit and risk limit concepts of radiological protection and safety from injury as shown in Figures 9.8 and 10.2. So far, though, the numerical values of *de minimis* and *de manifestis* risk have not been defined and we will consider that next. A point to note is that there is a lot of sensitivity about *de minimis* risk in particular, because sometimes even very small risks are perceived as undesirable and so the use of words like 'acceptable risk' may be challenged. For example, a typical response might be 'acceptable to whom?' You will learn more about this in Chapter 12, but for the time being, remember it is a sensitive matter. As the engineer Samuel Florman said of risk assessment, but which has wider resonance, 'Responsible experts in the field, however, consistently warn that risk assessment is a delicate tool that needs to be applied sparingly, not a machete to be flailed against the supposedly overgrown regulatory jungle' (Florman 1987).

2 It can be inferred that the vestiges of a consistent philosophy exist in the form of risk or dose limits and concepts like ALARA and ALARP which have a great deal in common. What differs most, perhaps, is the extent to which the existence of these concepts is recognized and understood in different professions, areas of application, and by the affected public.

Risk limits for carcinogenic substances in the environment

As noted above, although the utility of *de minimis* and *de manifestis* risk levels for hazardous substances has been identified, the actual corresponding risk levels so far have not been defined numerically. In fact, you have to dig quite deeply to discover what they might be. To this effect, in 1987, Curtis Travis and colleagues conducted a review of a large number of US federal regulatory decisions relating to the management of environmental carcinogens with a view to discovering if a consistent pattern existed in terms of those risk levels which were seen as requiring, or not requiring, regulatory action.

Activity 10.5

With reference to Figure 8.3, how would you describe the approach used by Travis and colleagues to discover society's position with regard to risks of environmental carcinogens?

Feedback

This is an example of a willingness-to-pay (WTP) revealed preference study based on regulatory/institutional decisions.

Travis et al. considered three measures of risk in their analysis. These were: (1) individual risk defined as the upper limit estimate of the probability that the most highly exposed individual in a population would develop cancer as a result of a lifetime of exposure; (2) the size of the population exposed; and (3) the population risk defined as the upper limit estimate of the number of additional annual incidences of cancer in the exposed population. Figure 10.4 shows the raw results, in terms of pre-regulatory levels of maximum individual risk, as obtained by Travis et al. (1987).

Log of individual risk

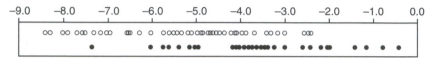

Figure 10.4 Pre-regulatory levels of maximum individual lifetime risk reviewed by federal agencies. O = agencies did not act to reduce public risk; ● = agencies acted to reduce public risk

Source: Travis et al. (1987)

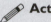 **Activity 10.6**

Examine Figure 10.4 carefully. What inferences can be drawn about the actions of regulators in response to different individual risk levels?

 Feedback

If you think quite carefully about it, there are two clear patterns in Figure 10.4. One is that for every chemical with an individual chronic risk of developing cancer above 4×10^{-3} (four chances in a thousand), a regulatory action was taken. Second, with one exception, no action was taken to reduce individual lifetime risk levels that were below 1 in 10^{-6}.

Travis et al. also examined the data to see if the size of the population exposed had an effect upon the level at which regulatory action was taken. Figure 10.5 shows the results. Note that population risk has been calculated by multiplying individual risk by population exposed and is expressed as cancer deaths per year.

 Activity 10.7

The following passage extracted from Travis et al. (1987) interprets the data in Figure 10.5. What does this tell you about the actual levels of *de manifestis* and *de minimis* risk for small populations, and how is the appropriateness of regulation for risks between these boundaries assessed?

📖 **Identification of *de manifestis* and *de minimis* levels**

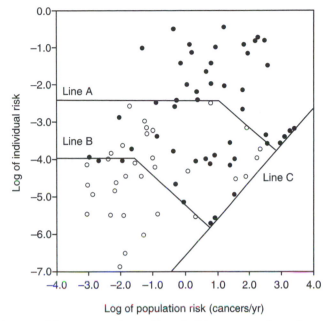

Key: ○ Agencies did not act to reduce public risk; ●Agencies acted to reduce public risk.

Figure 10.5 The effect of individual and population risk on whether or not risk posed by a chemical carcinogen in the environment is regulated or not

Source: Travis et al. (1987)

Line A of Figure 10.5 defines the *de manifestis* level: above this line, federal agencies always acted to reduce risk. For exposures resulting in small-population risk, the *de manifestis* level is approximately 4×10^{-3}. As population risk approaches 250 cancer deaths (which would occur in a population of 230 million as in the USA) the *de manifestis* level drops to about 3×10^{-4}. Line B shows the *de minimis* level. Below this line, no action has ever been taken to reduce risk. Line B indicates that for small-population effects, regulatory action was never taken for individual risk levels below 10^{-4}. For effects resulting from exposure of the entire US population, the level of acceptable risk drops to 10^{-6}. Line C is the area beyond which no data can fall. It is determined by the maximum population which can be exposed, 230 million in this case.

Figure 10.5 raises two questions. First, what justification is given by regulatory agencies for not regulating chemicals in the *de minimis* category of risk? Second, what justification is given for regulatory decisions involving chemicals in the region between the *de manifestis* and *de minimis* levels? The primary answer given to the first question is insignificant population risk. In relation to the second, analysis of regulatory decisions involving chemicals in the region between the *de manifestis* and *de minimis* levels indicates that cost-effectiveness is the primary determinant of regulation . . .

In the region between the *de manifestis* and *de minimis* levels, substances with risk reduction costs of less than $2 million per life saved were regulated; substances that cost more were not regulated. This conclusion is based on limited data, but it is consistent with EPA guidance suggesting that regulation is warranted if the cost per life saved does not exceed $1.5 million.

 Feedback

Travis et al. conclude that for small populations at risk the *de minimis* risk level is at about 10^{-4} lifetime risk of dying from cancer. If you consider that most people live for ~50 to 80 years, this is equivalent to an annual risk of from 10^{-5} to 10^{-6}, which is broadly consistent with the figures proposed for the Tolerability of Risk framework for safety from injury. Likewise, for small exposed populations, the *de manifestis* risk level is equivalent to ~10^{-4} per annum which is the maximum value assigned to public risks in the ToR framework. The appropriateness of taking action at intermediate risk levels appears to be judged by examining the cost per life saved and comparing against a yardstick of $1.5 million (at 1987 costs). This is clearly tantamount to the use of cost–benefit analysis and is consistent with the philosophy of welfare economics.

Risk limits for non-carcinogenic substances in the environment

Separate criteria are necessary for non-carcinogenic hazardous chemicals because they are assumed to have different dose–response relationships, specifically, a threshold form versus the LNT form hypothesized for carcinogens. Generally, the approach for non-carcinogens is that levels in the environment are considered to be *de minimis* if the reference dose (RfD) is not exceeded for intakes from all exposure pathways.

The following passage by Kocher (1996) describes how the US Environmental Protection Agency (EPA) establishes RfDs for different chemicals. You will recognize the approach from your reading of Chapter 5.

 Establishing RfDs for different chemicals

The EPA's approach to establishing the RfD for any noncarcinogen usually starts with an estimate of the no-observed-adverse-effects level (NOAEL), which is the highest dose delivered to humans or test animals for which there are no statistically or biologically significant increases in the frequency or severity of adverse health effects. With only a few exceptions (e.g. arsenic), the estimated NOAEL is based on animal data. As an alternative, if the NOAEL has not been established, the EPA starts with an estimate of the lowest-observed-adverse-effects level (LOAEL), which generally is higher than the NOAEL and is the lowest dose delivered at which significant health effects are induced. Thus, for any noncarcinogen, either the NOAEL or the LOAEL is used to define an assumed threshold for adverse health effects.

The EPA then establishes the RfD as a dose intended to be adequately protective of public health by applying several safety and uncertainty factors to the observed NOAEL or LOAEL, which take into account various sources of uncertainty in the data used to derive the NOAEL or LOAEL and in extrapolating the data from animals to humans. These safety and uncertainty factors generally include a factor of 10 to account for the variability in susceptibility in the general population, with the intent of protecting especially sensitive subpopulations (e.g. children and the elderly); a factor of 10 when extrapolating from animals to humans to account for the possible interspecies variability in susceptibility; a factor of 10 when a NOAEL is derived from a study involving sub-chronic exposures, rather than longer-term chronic exposures; and a factor of 10 when using a LOAEL rather than a NOAEL to account for the uncertainty in extrapolating from LOAELs to NOAELs. In addition, the EPA may apply a modifying factor to account for any other uncertainties and judgmental factors not addressed in the safety and uncertainty factors described above.

Thus, the RfD generally is intended to be well below any threshold for adverse health effects. In particular, when the RfD is based on animal studies, which usually is the case, its value generally is set at least a factor of 100 and sometimes more than a factor of 1000 below the threshold, as represented by the NOAEL or LOAEL.

There are two considerations indicating that RfDs are properly interpreted as upper bounds on de minimis doses for noncarcinogenic hazardous chemicals. The first is the use of large safety and uncertainty factors in deriving RfDs from observed thresholds for adverse health effects, as described above, which again are intended to ensure that doses to individual members of the public would be well below any thresholds. Indeed, because of the way RfDs are derived, there should be no evidence that doses somewhat above an RfD would cause any adverse health effects.

The second consideration is that RfDs are presumed to be sufficiently far below any thresholds for adverse health effects that action to reduce doses at levels below RfDs generally is not required by the EPA. That is, RfDs are used to distinguish between doses that are trivial and, thus, require no further consideration and doses that are sufficiently high that consideration must be given to the feasibility of dose reduction. However, as is the case with the upper bound on de minimis risk for carcinogens, reduction of doses above RfDs generally is required only to the extent practicable.

As a cautionary note, there are suggestions that exposures to toxic substances at RfD levels are not necessarily associated with minimal appreciable risk after lifetime inhalation or ingestion (e.g. Castorina and Woodruff 2003), despite the use of large safety margins.

Summary

Various systems are used to help policy makers make decisions about health, safety and environmental protection on a consistent basis. These systems have much in common, relying as they do on science and economics, and in this sense they are sometimes referred to as 'rational' models. They are used worldwide, but are none-theless not widely known, let alone understood outside of professional circles. The systems all aim to maximize the use of resources in the interest of the public good, while also providing safeguards so that distributional inequities (unfair risk apportionments) are, to some extent at least, contained.

References

Ball D and Goats G (1996). Risk management and consumer safety. International Journal for Consumer Safety 3(3): 111–24.
Castorina R and Woodruff T (2003) Assessment of potential risk levels associated with US EPA reference values. Environmental Health Perspectives 111(10): 1318–25.

Florman SC (1987) *The Civilized Engineer*. New York: St Martin's Press.

Green J (1997) *Risk and Misfortune: The Social Construction of Accidents*. London: UCL Press.

HSE (1988) *The Tolerability of Risk from Nuclear Power Stations*. London: HMSO.

HSE (2002) *Reducing Risk, Protecting People*. Sudbury: HSE Books.

Kocher DC (1996) *Criteria for Establishing de minimis Levels of Radionuclides and Hazardous Chemicals in the Environment*. Oak Ridge National Laboratory, Report No. ES/Er/TM–187.

Maritime and Coastguard Agency (2006) Safer lives, safer ships, cleaner seas. Available at: http://www.mcga.gov.uk/

Travis CC, Richter SS, Crouch AC, Wilson R and Klema ED (1987) Cancer risk management: a review of 132 federal regulatory decisions. *Environmental Science and Technology* 21: 415–20.

UK Cabinet Office (2002) *Risk: Improving Government's Capability to Handle Risk and Uncertainty*. London: HM Cabinet Office.

World Health Organization (2002) *Injury: A Leading Cause of the Global Burden of Disease 2000*. Geneva: WHO.

SECTION 4

Beyond the rational action approach

11 | An introduction to alternative theories of risk

Overview

Now that you have studied, in Sections 2 and 3, the dominant paradigm of environmental health policy making, it is necessary to consider some of the objections and counter-arguments. Policy making, by its nature, is controversial, and the best way to deal with this is, first, to understand why.

This section starts with a consideration of the now familiar policy tools of environmental risk assessment, Pareto optimization, and cost–benefit analysis, and how they are regarded by those who are familiar with them. Arguments and counter-arguments will be examined. You will find also that sociology actually provides a number of quite different perspectives on health risk, besides the (rational) model explored so far, which have different implications for policy formulation. In Chapters 12 and 13 you will look more closely at two of these, notably, the psychometric paradigm and cultural theory.

Learning objectives

By the end of this chapter, you will be better able to:

- **discuss the pros and cons of risk assessment and allied techniques as an aid to policy makers**
- **identify limitations of the techniques**
- **reflect on measures which might improve their acceptability.**

Key terms

Cultural theory A social theory that proposes that social responses to risks are determined by cultural belief patterns and not objective facts about risk.

Precautionary principle A principle that advocates the use of 'prudent' social policy in the absence of empirical evidence in an attempt to solve a problem.

Psychometric paradigm An approach to understanding public attitudes to different risks based on the use of quantitative techniques.

Rational actor paradigm (RAP) A sociological theory of human behaviour based on people acting as self-seeking individuals and maximizing their personal utility.

Challenges to the rational actor paradigm

So far in this book you have read about an approach to environmental health policy which is anchored in risk assessment, potential Pareto optimization (and hence neo-classical welfare economics), and calls upon allied techniques such as cost–benefit analysis even in applications involving public health. This is a particular approach which some theorists and sociologists describe as the rational actor paradigm (RAP). Most people acknowledge that RAP is a powerful and in many cases socially beneficial tool, but it is certainly not without its critics and it is at the very least important to understand their concerns.

What exactly is meant by RAP? RAP is a way of thinking that can be traced back to classical Greece and which gained in influence during the Italian Renaissance and the period in Europe (mainly in the eighteenth century) known as the Enlightenment. At the centre of this essentially Western world-view is the idea that humans are rational organisms and that the social world can be explained in terms of the interaction of humans as atomistic entities, rather like the natural world can be explained by the interaction of atoms. This world-view sees humans as rational beings motivated by pure self-interest and consciously evaluating alternative courses of action (Jaeger et al. 2001). Welfare economics, including willingness-to-pay methodologies, is reliant upon this assumption. Essentially, RAP is about maximization, or, as you have also discovered, 'optimization'.

However, sociologists, and others, argue that there is far more to life than that. It is different and more complicated. There now follows two abridged passages by leading sociologists Carlo Jaeger and colleagues, and Michiel Schwartz and Michael Thompson, which identify the nature of some of these concerns.

 Activity 11.1

While reading these extracts, think of what they might mean for the so-called RAP which you have studied in earlier chapters. In particular, consider the following questions:

1 What is the main point being made by each of the authors?
2 What are the implications for policy making?

 RAP and policy

Our main point here is that the realm of RAP has been extended beyond its scope to areas that cannot and should not be regarded as maximization or optimization problems. RAP assumes that individuals pursue the three requisite steps of decision making: option generation, evaluation of consequences, and selection of the most beneficial option. Without a doubt there are many social situations that can be described or at least simulated in such a fashion. There are many other situations, however, in which the model of decision making as an act of optimizing outcomes appears to be a weak descriptor for what actually happens, let alone for what the actors perceive to happen. Social reality becomes impoverished if all actions have only one common goal: to maximize or optimize one's utility. Balancing social relations, finding meaning within a culture, showing sympathy and empathy to others as well as being accepted or even loved by other individuals belong to a class of social phenomena that do not fit neatly into the iron rule of RAP theory. Individuals may behave in accordance with the means–end optimization process of RAP some of the time, but certainly not all of the time (Jaeger et al. 2001).

All policy debates revolve around *people* and *ideas*. Poverty, for instance, has to do with some people's lack of command over resources relative to their needs, and poverty policy has to do with the ideas of distributional justice that define a more desirable state of affairs (the policy goal) and with the ideas both of the processes by which poverty comes about and of the ways we can intervene in those processes to modify the outcomes (the instrumental means towards the policy goal). But some policy debates, the conventional wisdom tells us, revolve around *things* as well (nuclear power stations, chemical waste, drinking water quality, and so on), and it is this quality of 'thingness' that has been used to separate out technological decision making as a distinct kind of decision making, one in which the debate revolves around a technical and factual core that simply does not exist in other kinds of decision making.

It is with this starting point that we take issue. There is, we insist, no policy debate that is devoid of things, though, of course, some are more thing-ridden than others. Poverty policy, for instance, is not usually considered a part of technological decision making yet it is nevertheless much involved with things as well as with people and ideas. Nor are the facts concerning those things, and the uncertainties that often surround those facts, ever merely technical. They are every bit as value-driven as are any of the other interactions within this triangular interplay of people, ideas and things. Where others have assumed the interplay of just people and ideas to be the natural habitat of policy, and have then had to designate a special category of decision making for those environments where things are involved as well, we begin by assuming that this 'special case' is the normal (indeed, the inescapable) state of affairs, and then set out to explore the continuum of variation in policy debates as the relative contributions of these three essential elements – people, ideas and things – vary (Schwartz and Thompson 1990).

↻ Feedback

1. The main point being made by Carlo Jaeger et al. stems from the fact that RAP emerges from a theoretical basis which assumes that people behave in particular ways for particular reasons, but that this is only partially reflective of the truth. People are more than profit or utility maximizers. They aspire to (nobler) things which (for all we know) may have been instrumental in the survival of the human race.

2. It follows that, if the theoretical background is faulty, then a policy process derived from that theory may not reflect human aspirations. Were this so, it could spell trouble.

Michiel Schwartz and Michael Thompson are also concerned that policy debates which involve the more easily recognizable technical issues have, for no good reason, been shunted off into a distinct kind of decision making process (which we may identify with RAP). This process aspires not to be value-driven by relying upon facts, welfare economics, PPI and the like, but all of these actually involve values in some way or another. For example, the issue of distributional justice is not a part of neo-classical welfare economics, having been delegated by economists to philosophers and politicians, but the mere act of omitting it implies the making of a value decision.

This is not to say that these authors are necessarily antagonistic to the RAP approach, rather, that it has strengths and it has weaknesses too. Environmental health policy makers will want to understand this very clearly.

So what, then, are the main categories of criticism overall which have been levelled at risk assessment and the associated decision techniques as a tool for environmental health policy? The following extract from a paper by environmental scientist Ken Sexton (2000) provides a concise and useful summary under six headings, with responses.

 Critiques of risk assessment

Ethical critique

Because risk-based approaches fail to safeguard human health and the environment adequately they are ethically unacceptable. *Response*: the evidence suggests, to the contrary, that risk-based approaches have been largely successful in protecting people and environmental quality, and that their effectiveness will continue to improve over time.

Alternative paradigm critique

The 'Precautionary Principle' is preferable to the risk assessment paradigm because it places the burden of proof on the proponent of an activity, substance, or technology, rather than on the public. *Response*: decisions about burden of proof are value-based policy calls reflecting societal judgments. The fact is both paradigms require formalized risk assessment procedures to ensure adequate protection of human health and environmental quality.

Empirical critique

Valid risk estimates are precluded by large scientific uncertainties, which derive from both a scarcity of data (lack of knowledge) and limitations on our ability to interpret available data (lack of adequate understanding). *Response*: risk assessment provides a valuable framework for organizing and analyzing available scientific information and identifying key data gaps and methodological shortcomings, which can then be addressed through targeted research.

Methodological critique

Quantitative risk assessment focuses inappropriately on a single dimension (probability of specified harm) and therefore does not capture the most important dimensions of risk (knowledge, dread). *Response*: expert estimates of risk establish the foundation for scientifically sound decision making, and do not impede consideration of other relevant factors, including public perceptions and values.

Political critique

Despite claims that its goal is to produce more rational, science-based decisions, risk assessment is actually used as a smoke screen by those who want to ignore or trivialize certain risks. *Response*: the vast majority of proponents advocate use of formalized risk assessment because they believe it is an invaluable decision-making tool that contributes directly to more informed and more reasonable environmental decisions.

Procedural critique

Whether it is more rational, the process of relying exclusively on expert judgment to evaluate risks is not fair because citizens and communities have a right to participate in decisions directly affecting their health and well being. *Response*: it does not have to be one way or the other. An integrated approach, which involves the public in identifying and evaluating risks, is emerging as a middle-of-the-road alternative.

In reading the above extract, you will have discovered reference to two drivers for change which seek to turn RAP, and traditional risk assessment, into forms more universally acceptable to policy making. These are the reference to 'knowledge and dread' as dimensions of risk which must be considered, and to the desirability of public participation in health risk decision making. There is also reference to an alternative paradigm – the Precautionary Principle. In the remaining chapters you will read more about these developments. First, though, as a means of injecting some order into the process, it is helpful to consider a classification, by the sociologist Ortwin Renn, of the major sociological perspectives on risk.

Alternatives to RAP

Ortwin Renn's classification of sociological perspectives on risk is shown in Figure 11.1 (Renn 2005). The rational actor approach can be seen in the bottom-left

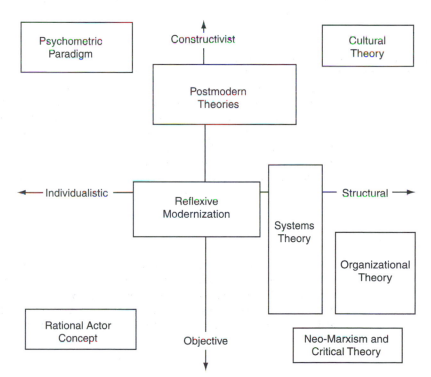

Figure 11.1 Major sociological perspectives on risk
Source: Reproduced with permission of Ortwin Renn (2005)

corner, and there are clearly a number of other models on offer also shown in the diagram. You will be reading about two of these in particular, the psychometric paradigm and cultural theory, in the following chapters. It is important to understand the meaning of the dimensions. This will become clearer when you have read about the other models, but a short explanation will be given here.

The horizontal axis ranges from individualistic to structural. This refers to the base unit of the model. In the case of RAP, this is an atomistic model for which the base unit is the individual. According to this model, society is made up of a myriad of individuals who independently try to maximize their personal utility. For this reason, RAP is located on the left of Figure 11.1. However, other theories take a different perspective. People are seen not to act individually but as part of a social group, a subculture or a society. Theories, like neo-Marxism and cultural theory, which explain risk behaviour from this perspective, are located on the right.

The vertical axis ranges from objective to constructivist. Whereas the objectivist concept implies that risk is an objective, measurable entity, which can be systematically prioritized, the constructivist concept denies this. Instead, it sees risks as 'socially constructed'. The social construction idea is based on the observation that people somehow agree to ignore most of the potential dangers around them, but interact so as to concentrate only on risks which they select for their attention for a variety of reasons (Douglas and Wildavsky 1983), even though these may carry a minimal actual risk. On this dimension, RAP clearly belongs at the bottom of this axis, being anchored in attempts to quantify risk, and hence its overall position is in the bottom-left corner of Figure 11.1.

In defence of cost–benefit analysis

In 1996, a group of leading American economists spoke out in defence of the use of benefit–cost analysis in policy decisions affecting the environment, health and safety (Arrow et al. 1996). They noted that the use of benefit–cost analysis in the fields of environmental protection, health and safety was controversial and sought to develop a consensus by setting out principles in a straightforward fashion. They advise that their pamphlet should be required reading for policy makers who wish to understand both the strengths and limitations of benefit–cost analysis in the development, design and implementation of policy.

 Activity 11.2

The key principles, from the perspective of environmental health policy, set out by Kenneth Arrow and colleagues (1996) are summarized below in two parts (some minor modifications have been made, but only to adapt them for the purposes of this book). In reading them, consider and make notes on the extent to which the principles address and deal with the criticisms identified earlier in this chapter.

Arrow's principles

1 Guidance for decision makers on using economic analysis to evaluate proposed policies

(a) A benefit–cost analysis is a useful way of organizing a comparison of the favourable and unfavourable effects of proposed policies.

(b) Economic analyses can be useful in designing regulatory strategies that achieve a desired goal at the lowest possible cost.

(c) Benefit–cost analysis should be required for all major regulatory (or policy) decisions.

(d) Policy makers should not be bound by a strict benefit–cost test, but should be required to consider available benefit–cost analyses. For regulations (or policies) whose expected costs far exceed expected benefits, a clear justification should be required.

2 Suggestions for improving the quality of economic analysis used in decision making

(a) While benefit–cost analysis should focus primarily on the overall relationship between benefits and costs, a good benefit–cost analysis will identify important distributional consequences of a policy.

(b) It is important to identify the incremental costs and benefits associated with different policies.

(c) Benefits and costs of proposed policies should be quantified wherever possible. Best estimates should be presented along with a description of uncertainties.

(d) Not all impacts of a decision can be quantified or expressed in dollar terms. Care should be taken to assure that quantitative factors do not dominate important qualitative factors in decision making.

(e) The more external review analyses receive, the better they are likely to be.

(f) A core set of economic assumptions should be used in calculating benefits and costs associated with environmental, health, and safety policies. Key variables include the discount rate, the value of reducing risks of dying and accidents, and the value associated with other improvements in health.

(g) Information should be presented clearly and succinctly. Transparency is necessary if benefit–cost analysis is to inform decision making.

(h) Whenever possible, values for monetizing benefits and costs should be based on trade-offs that individuals would make, either directly or, as is often the case, indirectly in labor, housing, or other markets.

(i) Given uncertainties in identifying the correct discount rate, it is appropriate to employ a range of rates.

Feedback

Principles 1(a) to 1(c) maintain the status quo, but 1(d) seemingly goes some way to addressing the critiques. Thus, it says, benefit–cost analysis (BCA) *should* be used, but *should not* be absolutely binding. And if the BCA shows a proposed policy to have a very poor benefit to cost ratio, then a good justification would be required if it were being recommended for implementation. This appears reasonable.

Principle 2(a) addresses head-on the distributional issue and is a clear signal that this is important. 2(c) and 2(i) are important in that they stress the need to identify uncertainties, something which has not been a strong point in economics, and test their effect upon policy options. 2(d) is very important regarding the critiques – many concerns that people have about policies will relate to aspects that can only be described qualitatively. There has long been a fear that analyses that include quantitative and qualitative factors will tend to devalue the qualitative ones. Whether this can be achieved in practice, however, remains to be seen. 2(e) and 2(g) are helpful in that they potentially open up the analysis so that there can be wider scrutiny. This is a small step in the direction of the opposition. Principles 2(f) and 2(h), however, which imply adherence to contingent valuation, look set to continue to be regions of contention.

Summary

The formulation of anything as important, and contentious, as environmental health policy requires a professional approach, and true professionalism requires an understanding of the strengths and limitations of your position. Environmental health risk assessment is a comparatively young discipline and it should be no surprise therefore if it is imperfect. In this chapter you have discovered a range of criticisms, and some responses, by different disciplines including, notably, sociology. This provides a foundation for looking more closely at some alternative explanations of society's response to risk with which environmental health policy makers need to be familiar.

References

Arrow KJ et al. (1996) *Benefit–Cost Analysis in Environmental, Health, and Safety Regulation: A Statement of Principles*. Annapolis: The Annapolis Center.

Douglas M and Wildavsky A (1983) *Risk and Culture*. Berkeley, CA: University of California Press.

Jaeger CC, Renn O and Rosa EA (2001) *Risk, Uncertainty and Rational Action*. London: Earthscan.

Renn O (2005) personal communication. An earlier version appeared in Krimsky S and Golding G (eds) (1992), *Social Theories of Risk*, chapter 3. Westport, CT: Praeger.

Schwartz M and Thompson M (1990) *Divided We Stand: Redefining Politics, Technology and Social Choice*. New York: Harvester Wheatsheaf.

Sexton K (2000) Socioeconomic and racial disparities in environmental health: is risk assessment part of the problem or part of the solution? *Human and Ecological Risk Assessment* 6(4): 561–74.

12 Risk perception and the psychometric paradigm

Overview

In Chapter 11 you were introduced to the existence of some alternative theories of risk, besides the 'rational' model, which offer different explanations of how people react to and evaluate risk. Two of these will now be discussed in more detail. The first, dealt with in this chapter, is the psychometric paradigm and its antecedents. Referring back to Figure 11.1 you will see that this perspective, being located in the upper left quadrant, is based on the subjective views of individuals. Simply put, it is about how risks are *perceived* by *individuals*. An understanding of the public perception of risk is supremely important for environmental health policy makers for several reasons. Perhaps most important is that without it you might find it very difficult to implement policies.

Learning objectives

By the end of this chapter, you will be better able to:

- describe the contribution of psychology to the understanding of risk perception
- understand why the public and experts often feel differently about risk
- discuss two different ways in which the brain makes decisions
- identify qualitative aspects of hazards which affect the response of the public and therefore may be important to environmental health policy makers.

Key terms

Affect The automatic feeling of goodness or badness generated in response to some event.

Experiential learning Learning from experience.

Psychometrics The science of psychological measurement.

Risk aversion Here, a precautionary attitude towards risk taking.

Stakeholder An individual or group with a substantive interest in an issue (i.e. interest group), including those with some role in making a decision or its execution.

Why an understanding of risk perception is important

In the early days, by which is meant until some 30 years ago, it was common practice for risk decisions to be made by specialists who frequently saw little need to engage with those who would be affected. As time passed, this normally well-meaning but autocratic approach ran into increasing difficulty. Decisions made according to the so-called rules of 'rational decision making' were increasingly challenged by parties who had an interest in policy choices.

Table 12.1, based on information from the Centre for Environmental Justice in Sri Lanka in 2006, illustrates the breadth of issues which can give rise to controversy in just one part of the world. There are numerous other examples worldwide where the public, employees, and other stakeholders have felt it necessary to raise issues and even challenge risk decisions by professionals or governments. The consequences can be important – they might derail a programme aimed at improving public health, incur significant costs, or deter innovation. This is not to imply that these challenges to authority are necessarily wrong or unjustified. Without needing to take sides, it is clear that perceptions of risk do have immense consequences for society, just as they do for individuals. Environmental health policy makers therefore need to understand why this is so in order to have any prospect of resolving these issues.

Table 12.1 An example of environmental and health issues causing current concern in one region of the world, Sri Lanka

The issue	Nature of the concern
100 metre no construction zone in the coastal belt (a tsunami counter-measure)	Public unrest
The Sri Lankan civil war	No studies of the environmental consequences
Genetically modified food	Uncertainty over risks and benefits
Sulphur dioxide level in Columbo	Effect on sensitive groups
Menik Ganga River diversion	Water reduction for Yala and Kataragama villages
Persistent organic pollutants: (aldrin, dieldrin, DDT, chlordane, endrin, heptachlor, mirex, toxaphene, hexachlorobenzene, PCBs, dioxins, furans)	Cancer and other health effects
Incineration	Waste of resources and contamination
Uncontrolled logging	Conservation
Human–elephant conflict leading to 150 to 200 elephant deaths per year	Public concern
900 MW coal-fired power station to be built at Kalpitiya	Pollution
Columbo to Kandy highway	Will relocate many families and destroy paddy fields

Source: Based on the Sri Lanka Centre for Environmental Justice (2006)

Activity 12.1

Identify from your own experience (or from what you have seen in your local media), two issues where different perceptions of environmental health risk have resulted in controversy. What reasons can you think of that might underlie these conflicts?

 Feedback

You should have no difficulty in responding to the first question because the range of possibilities is immense. Of the second question, it can be said that controversies may be ignited by anything from different objectives, values, or perceptions of risk held by affected groups, and perhaps least likely but still plausible, disputes over technical assessments of risk. Or it may be that there has been a lack of political process in the form of consultation and communication.

Early studies of risk perception

In 1969, the American scientist Chauncey Starr authored what is now seen as a landmark paper that compared the benefits of selected technological activities with one particular cost, namely, the cost of accidental deaths associated with the activity. His aim was to find if there was a relationship between the level of risk of an activity which society would tolerate and its benefits. He used as examples a number of accepted activities, such as the use of motor vehicles, electricity generation, etc. (Starr 1969). Referring back to Figure 8.3, you should be able to identify this as an example of the 'revealed preference – individual choice – consumer market' method.

Starr concluded that the public is willing to accept 'voluntary' risks that are roughly 1,000 times greater than 'involuntary' risks giving the same benefit. He also concluded that the acceptability of risk appeared to depend on the benefits (real or imagined) of the activity. These findings seem eminently sensible. Yet these factors might not have been acknowledged in a strictly 'rational' (as defined earlier) decision making process.

Further influential research of a quite different nature was reported by Tversky and Kahneman in 1974, who found that when people are confronted with large amounts of information on some topic and have to form an opinion, they use mental short cuts, known as 'cognitive *heuristics*'. These help simplify information and reduce the amount of mental effort and time required to make a decision. Every time you cross a road you have to make a risk decision almost instantaneously. The use of heuristics focuses attention on the most prominent issue of the moment. A second factor they discovered was that of '*availability*'. That is, if you have an available image in your mind which relates to the issue in hand, it will influence your decision. Available images can be very powerful and long-lasting – see Figure 12.1.

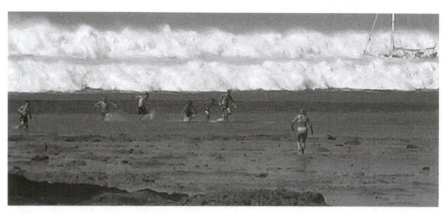

Figure 12.1 Anyone witnessing this scene of people fleeing for their lives from a tsunami would be likely to retain a vivid image in their memory.

 Activity 12.2

1   What available images do you personally recall that influence your decisions?
2   What available images can you think of which have influenced societal decisions?
3   Is the effect of these available images on decisions beneficial?

 Feedback

1 Available images come in many shapes and forms, depending upon your experiences. They may be of happy associations, or of frightening events, as in Figure 12.1.

2 Images of the December 2005 tsunami have encouraged society to set up a seismic monitoring network in the Indian Ocean, even though these events are exceedingly rare.

3 Psychologists believe that available images are one of the ways in which human beings have been able to make decisions and to survive. However, they can be misleading and where important decisions are being made, it would be inadvisable to be over-reliant upon them. Analysis, too, should be used.

Differing perceptions of risk

In the 1970s, Sarah Lichtenstein and her co-workers decided to take forward Starr's work using quantitative expressed preference techniques. They did this by asking ordinary people to estimate the risk of dying from a wide range of causes (e.g. heart disease, cancer, botulism, tornadoes, etc.) and comparing their answers against actual risk as deduced from official statistics. They also put the same questions to experts.

ordinary people to estimate the risk of dying from a wide range of causes (e.g. heart disease, cancer, botulism, tornadoes, etc.) and comparing their answers against actual risk as deduced from official statistics. They also put the same questions to experts.

The results of the first part of this work are found in Figure 12.2. This shows (vertical axis) the annual number of deaths in the USA, where the study was made, as estimated by a sample of Americans, versus actual statistical estimates (horizontal axis). The important thing about this graph is that if the judgements of probability were accurate, they would fall on the straight line at 45 degrees to each axis, but they don't. It looks instead as if the frequency of rare events is being overestimated and that of common events underestimated. The reason why the probability of rare events is overestimated might in part be down to the 'availability heuristic' if images of these events have lodged in the memory.

The results of the second part of this study, the comparison of public assessments of risk with those of experts, are summarized in Figure 12.3. It can be seen (from the slopes of the lines) that the expert ratings are more closely associated with the actual risk of death. Note that it is not said that the expert ratings are more 'accurate'. The reason for this will become apparent shortly.

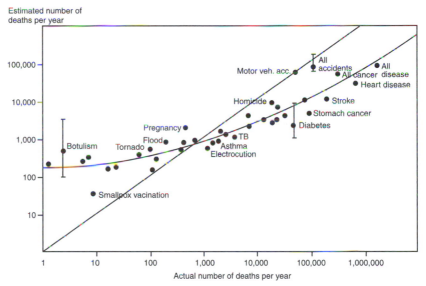

Figure 12.2 The judged versus actual risk of particular harms

Source: Lichtenstein et al. (1978)

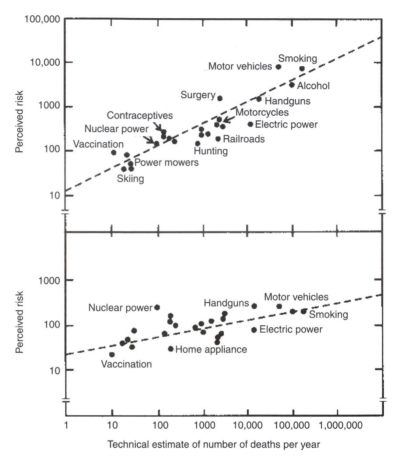

Figure 12.3 The top graph compares expert perceived ratings of risk against technical estimates and the bottom graph does the same for lay people. Note that the experts' ratings are more closely associated with actual fatality rates.

Source: Slovic (2000)

✎ Activity 12.3

The above difference between expert and lay estimations of risk is often quoted and has been very influential. It has led some people to propose that the lay public are rather ignorant about risk and that what is needed is education so that they think like experts. What do you think of this proposition?

↻ Feedback

This is a controversial area which we will discuss in more detail later. There is truth in the proposition that experts are more knowledgeable about the numerical risks posed by hazards than the public. But on the other hand, the public may have legitimate concerns which are not encapsulated by the experts' opinions where these are based solely upon considerations of risk magnitude.

The multi-dimensional nature of hazards

The above question, over the difference between expert and lay perceptions of risk, was reframed by the American psychologist Paul Slovic and co-workers. What, they asked, do non-experts actually mean when they say that some situation or some activity is risky? Further research showed that whereas experts, in rating risks, were primarily focusing on associated fatality rates, lay people had a much wider interpretation of risk. This was demonstrated by asking lay people to rate hazards against a number of qualitative dimensions besides pure risk of harm. Figure 12.4 shows the results for one pair of hazards, both being sources of ionizing radiation, and hence posing a risk of cancer. What is clear is that the lay perceptions of these two hazards are quite different in terms of these qualitative characteristics. If lay people were incorporating factors of this kind into their overall rating of hazards, this could explain the differences between public and expert opinion in Figure 12.3.

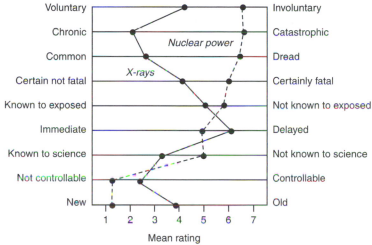

Figure 12.4 Qualitative characteristics of perceived risk for two hazards giving rise to ionizing radiation

Note: Each profile is based on subjective ratings against nine dimensions on a seven-point scale.

Source: Slovic (2000)

Activity 12.4

Do your own rating on a seven-point scale of two quite different hazards with which you are familiar against the following five qualitative characteristics:

1 Voluntary (1) to involuntary (7).
2 Familiar (1) to unfamiliar (7).
3 Not fatal (1) to fatal (7).
4 You know when you are exposed (1) to you don't know (7).
5 It is understood by science (1) to it is not understood (7).

What conclusion do you draw about the importance of these characteristics in your overall assessment of the relative risk?

Feedback

If you allow yourself to think about the hazards in general terms you will probably find, if the hazards are sufficiently different, that the pattern of scoring differs significantly against the five criteria. Whether or not this influences your decision about their overall relative importance will depend upon your perspective. For many people, factors like these are influential.

The psychometric paradigm

Paul Slovic and his co-workers have greatly extended their work since those early days and it has by now been replicated in countries all around the world. To understand why some hazards are perceived as more risky than others they employed the 'psychometric paradigm' where psychometrics is a term referring to the measurement of mental attitudes. This used a questionnaire which asked participants to rate a selection of hazards against the following 15 characteristics:

- whether observable or not;
- whether known to those exposed;
- whether effects were delayed (a reference to carcinogens and similar hazards);
- whether a new risk;
- whether known to science;
- whether controllable;
- whether dreaded;
- whether globally catastrophic;
- whether fatal;
- whether equitable;
- whether affecting an individual;
- whether posing a risk to future generations;
- whether not easily reduced;
- whether the risk was increasing;
- whether voluntarily taken.

The methodology is in fact very similar to the one you used in Activity 12.4. A typical question was: 'How do you rate this hazard (e.g. chemical contamination of river water) in terms of its voluntariness? Give a score from 1 to 7, where 1 means it is entirely voluntary to 7 meaning it is entirely involuntary.' Participants were also asked to rate the overall perceived risk of each hazard. The term 'risk' was left deliberately vague, so that participants could interpret it as they wished.

Slovic and co-workers found that each hazard had its own unique profile when scored against these attributes (such as X-rays and nuclear power in Figure 12.4). Because it is not possible to display these results in 15 dimensions, a statistical method called Factor Analysis was used to simplify the results. It turned out that many of the qualitative characteristics were closely inter-related. For example, a hazard such as riding a bicycle was seen as both voluntary and individual, and one such as genetic modification of crops was regarded as a new risk and unknown to science. Factor analysis showed that there were two dominant composite factors in operation which explained most of the differences in perception of the hazards. Factor 1 (referred to as known–unknown risk) was made up of the first five characteristics on the above list, and Factor 2 (referred to as 'dread' risk) was made up of the remainder.

In the original work, participants were asked to rate 81 hazards against these 15 dimensions and after Factor analysis the result shown in Figure 12.5 was obtained.

What does Figure 12.5 tell us? Overall, the higher a hazard's score on the Dread dimension in particular, the higher is its perceived risk. Hazards scoring highly on both the Dread and Unknown dimensions (those in the top-right quadrant of Figure 12.5) were of most concern for the public who wanted to see these risks reduced and strictly regulated. Experts, on the other hand, might not agree with this rating of risk, preferring to think simply about the expected value of the risk and the probability of actual harm. Hazards appearing in the lower-left quadrant, like bicycles and trampolines, are of less public concern, apparently because they are familiar and not associated with any of the components of dread. Of course, experts would still associate things like riding bicycles with risk, but the public, because of the qualitative factors, would tend to be less concerned about them and therefore rate them as less important.

The affect heuristic

Recently psychologists have begun to pursue a further line of inquiry into how we make choices. This is known as 'the affect heuristic', where 'affect' refers to the specific quality of goodness or badness which you experience as a feeling (with or without consciousness) when presented with some object or situation. Affective responses occur very quickly and automatically. Images like those in Figure 12.1, for example, automatically generate affective responses, some positive and some negative.

In Section 3 of this book we discussed rationalistic decision processes, based on cognitive thought processes, rather than upon affect-driven processes. Note that the dictionary defines cognition as 'conceiving of something by mental processes as distinct from emotion and volition'. Both of these processes occur in the brain, so it's as if the brain has two ways of arriving at decisions (no doubt this will turn out to be an over-simplification). Most of the risk decisions we have to make have to be made quickly, hence relying on what might be called an instinctive reaction. This need would favour, even require, the use of the affect heuristic because it is quick. The other approach is analytic – with time to spare, we may spend much time analysing the pros and cons of alternative strategies.

Activity 12.5

Give an example of a decision you have made based on the affect heuristic and one based on a cognitive process.

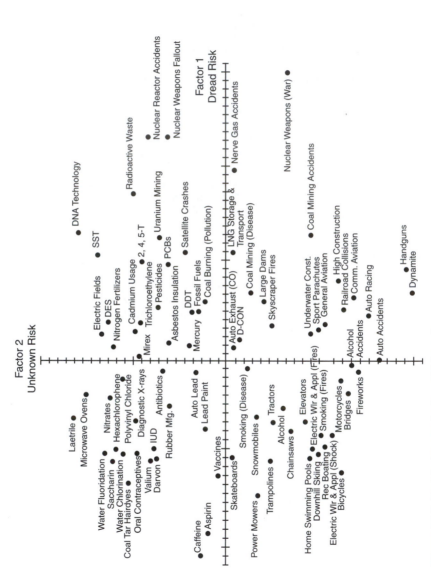

Figure 12.5 Slovic's characterization of 81 hazards

Source: Slovic (2000)

Feedback

As is often said, 'Is it your heart or your head that makes decisions?' The heart is associated with emotion and intuition, and the head with analysis and wisdom. Human beings rely upon both. You should not find it difficult to answer this question.

Despite the emphasis within organizations upon the cognitive-rationalistic approach to decision making, the existence of affect and its contribution to cognitive decision processes have actually been known and exploited, not always for good, throughout the ages.

Epstein (1994) has summed up the situation very clearly:

There is no dearth of evidence in everyday life that people apprehend reality in two fundamentally different ways, one variously labelled intuitive, automatic, natural, non-verbal, narrative, and experiential, and the other analytical, deliberative, verbal, and rational.

The rational system is a deliberative, analytic system that functions by way of established rules of logic and evidence (e.g. probability theory). The experiential system encodes reality in images, metaphors, and narratives to which affective feelings have become attached.

This intuitive–experiential system of decision making to which Epstein refers is intimately associated with affect. It is believed to work as follows: when you encounter an emotionally significant event you automatically search your memory for similar events including their emotional accompaniments. If the feelings generated are pleasant, actions to reproduce the feelings are activated, and vice versa.

While there is a growing belief that cognitive heuristics, including the affect heuristic, are important aids to decision making, it is also felt that too much or too little affect can do disturbing things to your decision making processes. For example, there is evidence that the affect heuristic responds poorly to numerical information and this can have very real consequences in decision settings where resources need to be allocated.

Paul Slovic (2000) warns that:

the affect heuristic enables us to be rational actors in many important situations. But not in all situations. It works beautifully when our experience enables us to anticipate accurately how we will like the consequences of our decisions. It fails miserably when the consequences turn out to be much different in character than we anticipated.

Some difficulties of experiential learning

The affect heuristic is reliant upon experiential learning. This type of learning is and has been important for human survival but, like rational thinking, is vulnerable to various biases and shortcomings. Richard Eiser (2004) describes an example wherein a doctor is faced with a patient expressing some symptoms of potentially serious disease. Suppose a treatment is available which would benefit a patient who truly has the disease. The doctor has to decide whether to treat or not and may elect to do so on the basis of personal clinical experience. Now she may prefer to err on the side of safety and prescribe the treatment. This would lead to a situation in which experience of treating patients by some medical intervention was gained. However, the feedback which the doctor receives from this decision is selective, because the results of not treating the patient are unknown. For example, it could be that the symptoms would have gone away of their own accord. However, had this happened and the patient had been prescribed drugs, say, the doctor's belief in the efficacy of the drugs would have been falsely strengthened.

If the drugs are inexpensive and have no adverse effects, this might not matter. But suppose the treatment also has negative side-effects (as many do). Then the reliance on personal experience could lead to unnecessary prescription. In fact, there are four possibilities as shown in Table 12.2. A risk-averse doctor is likely to treat and gain experience of treated patients, but is less likely to have experience of patients who do not receive the treatment, leading to biased decision making.

As Eiser (2004) points out, this is a general problem in risk decision making where we rely upon experience. False alarms and risk aversion may be a consequence of the incomplete feedback we receive from everyday experiences. We only witness the consequences of our actions and not the alternatives.

Another difficulty with experiential learning is that in many situations feedback following some decision may be delayed. This has several implications. One is that causal pathways may be hidden. An example is the link between asbestos exposure and mesothelioma. Asbestos was used because of its valuable properties, some aimed at reducing risks, but knowledge and experience of long-term effects like mesothelioma were lacking and it was not until much later that causality between asbestos exposure and mesothelioma was determined. Likewise, the emission of carbon dioxide into the atmosphere was for centuries not a source of worry, but science now tells us it is linked to climate change.

Eiser (2004) also identifies the problem of over-generalization, or stigmatization. Because individual experiences are limited, particularly in the context of systems that operate relatively safely, we also rely on experiences of other people and news reports. Was the widely reported Chernobyl disaster, for example, peculiar to that type of nuclear reactor and the way it was managed, or does it represent an inherent problem of nuclear power generation? The affective and emotional associations of

Table 12.2 Decision consequences of medical diagnosis

Actual status of patient	Doctor's diagnosis	
	Disease present, prescribe treatment	Disease absent, no treatment prescribed
Disease present	True positive Correct diagnosis Appropriate treatment	False negative Incorrect diagnosis Failure to treat
Healthy, no disease	False positive Incorrect diagnosis Inappropriate treatment	True negative Correct diagnosis Unnecessary treatment avoided

Source: Eiser (2004)

that event are powerful, but very few of us understand the full, and still emerging, story and thus, in forming an opinion on the basis of Chernobyl, we may over-generalize.

Eiser's model of risk perception

Eiser has produced a helpful summary model of what you have read here about risk perception and the way in which the brain makes decisions (Figure 12.6). In this model, risk perception starts with some event which triggers memories and/or emotional reactions (affect heuristic). These result in an initial interpretation of the event in a relatively automatic way. At the same time, if the event is public and others experience it too, it will trigger responses which might lead to social reinforcement.

At this point, it may be that the individual will commence a more measured evaluation of the event by use of cognitive heuristics. Further information will also be received from experts which will be assessed for trustworthiness as well as meaning. These estimations, derived from the affect and cognitive heuristics, will then somehow be combined into a summary.

Individuals will then decide what to do. However, if they decide to treat the danger as real and avoid it, they will often not actually know if the danger was real (because they avoided it) nor if their actions were effective. Thus, there may be no evidence in the way of feedback so the apparent need for the possibly unnecessary action will be strengthened along with a potential increase in risk aversive tendencies. Alternatively, a decision to treat the situation as safe and approach the potential risk will provide the individual with useful feedback about the correctness of the decision, so updating experience and enhancing future judgement capabilities. However, the possibility will still exist that the feedback is misinterpreted, especially if it is inconsistent or delayed.

Activity 12.6

The work of Slovic and his colleagues demonstrates that public concerns about environmental hazards have, after all, a rational basis if you accept that factors such as 'dread' and 'voluntariness' are legitimate issues, and that affect-based choices may also have validity. Write down your thoughts on the implications of this for environmental health policy makers.

Feedback

The matter is far from simple. Policy makers will, on the one hand, feel compelled to maximize public health gains which implies a strictly rational decision making process. On the other hand, public concerns should be heeded in a democracy, but if this means allocating extra resources to an issue which is really a low priority in health terms, lives will be lost. The issue is further complicated by the fact that failure to legitimize public concerns may place obstacles in the way of purely rational policies, even though these would do the most good.

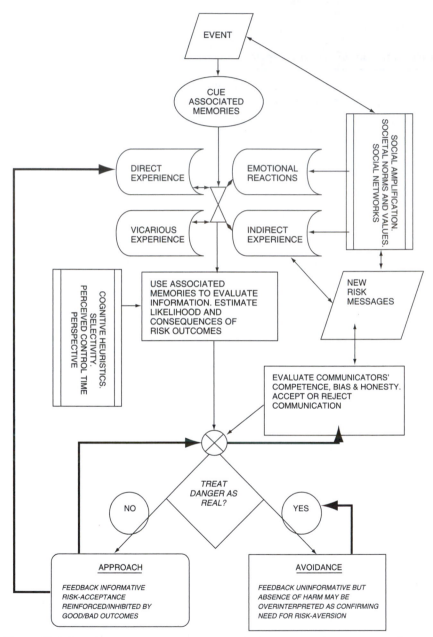

Figure 12.6 Flowchart representing processes involved in assessing the presence or absence of a risk

Source: Eiser (2004)

Summary

Research into risk perception points to two ways by which the brain makes decisions; either on the basis of rational analytic processes or affective response. The prevailing view is that both processes are necessary, one providing a check on the other. Research also reveals that the public tend to view risk in a more complex way than experts. Many qualitative factors contribute to the public perception of risk, whereas experts tend to rely upon rational, analytic assessments which in turn focus on the one-dimensional probability of actual harm. It is implied that if the public disagree with experts over the importance of a hazard, that this is not necessarily down to lack of knowledge (though this is possible), but may be because they have a 'richer' understanding of the meaning of risk.

References

Eiser RJ (2004) *The Public Perception of Risk*. London: Office of Science and Technology.

Epstein S (1994) Integration of the cognitive and psychodynamic unconscious, *American Psychologist*, 49: 709–24.

Lichtenstein S et al. (1978) The judged versus actual risk of particular harms. *Journal of American Psychology* 4: 551–78.

Slovic P (2000) *The Perception of Risk*. London: Earthscan.

Starr C (1969) Social benefits versus technological risk: what is our society willing to pay for safety? *Science* 165: 1232–8.

Tversky A and Kahneman D (1974) Judgment under uncertainty, *Science* 185: 1124–31.

Cultural theory

Overview

While the psychometric paradigm has deepened the understanding of risk controversies considerably, it suffers from the same micro-orientation as does RAP. For
this reason, cultural theory takes a very different approach in its attempt to understand why people perceive and react to risk the way they do. Unlike RAP and the
psychometric paradigm, it starts out with the supposition that people have one
of four different rationalities. Depending upon their 'choice' of rationality, they
will react differently to the risks which they encounter. Because cultural theory
permits this diversity, it is useful in understanding why risk issues are often debated
and even contentious, for if four different rationalities exist, then four different
interpretations of the same situation must be expected. This message can be very
troubling for decision makers, who normally are seeking a single interpretation of
the 'facts', and a unique and uncontested solution. However, the insights gained
from cultural theory are nonetheless very useful for decision makers, including
environmental health policy advisers, who will inevitably encounter a diversity of
responses to environmental health issues and must therefore be prepared, like it or
not, for a less than straightforward existence.

Learning objectives

By the end of this chapter, you will be better able to:

- **describe a third and radically different sociological model of risk**
- **recognize how it provides explanations of why environmental policy issues
  are often controversial**
- **discuss the implications for environmental health policy makers.**

Key terms

Objectivism The idea that risks can be measured and that we can distinguish between their real
magnitude and what people variously and perhaps erroneously believe them to be.

Relativism An extreme doctrine in which anyone's opinion is as good as anyone else's.

Social constructivism This approach to knowledge denies the existence of reality prior to
human engagement and the validity of 'truth' in the sense of a corresponding representation of
reality. Instead, it poses that reality is whatever is known, and that all knowledge is socially
produced. Constructivism can thus lead to relativism, as it allows no distinction between true
and untrue statements.

Where the story of cultural theory commenced

The story begins, or at least one thread of it, with natural science; the study of ecosystem management to be precise, which, by chance, is not a far cry from environmental health. From this work emerged the idea that all institutions (or, for that matter, policy makers), faced with exactly the same kind of situation, invariably adopted strategies based upon one of four different interpretations of the stability of the ecosystem (or policy issue) with which they were concerned. A further contention is that these four world-views, as we can call them, can be observed in numerous walks of life besides ecosystem management, certainly including environmental health policy formulation.

Activity 13.1

Read the following abridged account by the geographer John Adams (1995) of what are called the four 'myths of nature', corresponding to the four world-views mentioned above, each of which is said to capture *some* essence of human experience and wisdom.

1　Observe that the myths of nature are clearly depicted by the simple model of a ball in one of four possible landscapes as in Figure 13.1.
2　Think of an example of an environmental health issue which is managed according to each of these four myths or world-views.
3　How might the world-views help understand environmental health controversies?

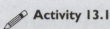 The four 'myths of nature'

Nature capricious

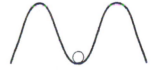

Nature perverse/tolerant

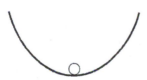

Nature benign

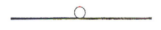

Nature ephemeral

Figure 13.1 The four myths of nature

Source: Adams (1995)

Nature benign: nature, according to this myth, is predictable, bountiful, robust, stable, and forgiving of any insults humankind might inflict upon it; however violently it might be shaken, the ball comes safely to rest in the bottom of the basin. Nature is the benign context of human activity, not something that needs to be managed. The management style associated with this myth is therefore relaxed, non-interventionist, *laissez-faire*.

Nature ephemeral: here nature is fragile, precarious and unforgiving. It is in danger of being provoked by human carelessness into catastrophic collapse. The objective of environmental management is the protection of nature from humans. People, the myth insists, must tread lightly on the Earth. The guiding management rule is the *precautionary principle*.

Nature perverse/tolerant: this is a combination of modified versions of the first two myths. Within limits, nature can be relied upon to behave predictably. It is forgiving of modest shocks to the system, but care must be taken not to knock the ball over the rim. Regulation is required to prevent major excesses, while leaving the system to look after itself in minor matters. This is the ecologist's equivalent of a mixed-economy model. The manager's style is *interventionist*.

Nature capricious: nature is unpredictable. The appropriate management strategy is again *laissez-faire*, in the sense that there is no point to management. Where adherents to the myth of 'nature benign' trust nature to be kind and generous, the believer in 'nature capricious' is agnostic; the future may turn out well or badly, but in any event it is beyond his control. The non-manager's motto is *que sera sera*.

Feedback

1 It should be clear that the world-view 'nature is benign' can be represented by a ball in a deep bucket. However hard you whack it, it will never escape. On the other hand, if you believe in 'nature perverse/tolerant' (which should sound familiar and remind you of ALARP/ALARA and the philosophy that risks, up to a point, are tolerable), a ball in a modestly deep bucket is what you have. In 'nature ephemeral' the ball is clearly delicately poised, and 'nature capricious' is like a marble on a flat surface – it rolls wherever it likes and is unpredictable.

2 Examples abound, but here are a few. For nature perverse/tolerant you might think of the general approach to the management of human exposure to toxic chemicals. Providing dose is managed so as to be below a certain threshold, then it is presumed that there is no harm. For nature benign, you might think of the past attitude of some industries and many nations to global carbon dioxide emissions. The atmosphere was deemed to be so large as to be beyond significant influence by humankind. For nature ephemeral, those who maintain that there are no 'safe' limits for, say, radiation exposure, adhere to this world-view. And, finally, for nature capricious, if you believe that some health conditions are induced by supernatural causes, or by events just too complicated to understand or control, then they would fit this model.

3 The world-views all exist at the same time. For every issue that you can identify, you will find some people who adhere to each world-view. In the case of personal injuries,

for example, some people believe that they are caused by accidents and are beyond control, and you might say that they subscribe to the world-view 'nature capricious'. Others believe, however, that accidents can and should be eliminated, even to the extent that the word 'accident' should no longer be used. These people could be aligned with a 'nature ephemeral' ideology, because their belief is that accidents are so serious that you would strive to eliminate them. Yet others, who have a 'nature benign' perspective, believe that the world is a hard place, and that sometimes we must expect to be injured in the quest for personal fulfilment. These people see nature as essentially benign in that it is not out to get them, but to be exploited, and for them, risks must be accepted and 'he who dares wins'. Finally, most professionals working in injury 'control', as they might call it, are trying to reduce injury risk, but only until as low as reasonably practicable (ALARP) – they are applying a nature perverse/tolerant model. In this way, cultural theory offers an insight into why these four very different ideas about, in this case, injury control, co-exist.

The understanding and utility of the above 'cultural theory' have also developed along another route by anthropologist Mary Douglas and her co-workers (Douglas 1985). They concluded that people's social relationships could also be classified into four types, and that these coincided neatly with the world-views in Figure 13.1.

Activity 13.2

In reading the following passage adapted from Schwartz and Thompson (1990), which outlines the thinking which gave rise to the identification of these four types of rationality (which are given the names 'hierarchist', 'egalitarian', 'individualist', and 'fatalist'), ask yourself if these four 'archetypes' really exist. It might help if you try to think of examples of types of people who seemingly fit these descriptions, and do you fit in there?

Four archetypes of rationality

The typology (developed by Mary Douglas and colleagues) is based on two central and eternal questions of human existence: 'who am I?' and 'how should I behave?' Personal identity (the first question), it is argued, is determined by individuals' relationships to *groups*. Those who belong to a strong group – a collective that makes decisions binding on all members – will see themselves very differently to those who have weak ties with others and therefore make choices that bind only themselves. Behaviour (the second question) is shaped by the extent of the social prescriptions (in Figure 13.2, this is the so-called '*grid*' dimension) that an individual is subject to: a spectrum which runs from the free spirit to the tightly constrained. These two 'dimensions of sociality', as it is called, generate four basic forms of social relationship, as set out in Figure 13.2.

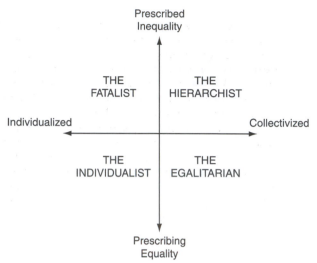

Figure 13.2 The four myths of human nature
Source: Adams (1995)

↻ **Feedback**

In some senses at least, these archetypes, with their associated ways of operating, can be observed throughout any society and at any level. Individualists, for example, can be likened to individual street or market traders who seek out the freedom to bid for and bargain with their wares, and for whom the important issue is their ability to 'make the books balance'. In contrast, hierarchists belong to orderly social groups who attempt to manage things according to established rules. You might find them in places ranging from offices, to government bureaucracies, to the organized religions, or the army. Egalitarians, in contrast, are characterized by a sense of community but with a tendency to be critical of both the status quo (loved by the hierarchist) and the unrestricted freedom and its impugned lack of collective responsibility (of the individualist). In the environmental arena, members of the Green pressure groups are often felt to be egalitarian in outlook. But not everyone who is unconnected to organized social groups can be described as an individualist, since that would mean they had freedom to act. In fact, they might be in a very weak position to influence events and thus their situation is more akin to one of fatalism, for they cannot influence the things which will happen to them.

Having encountered the four myths of nature (world-views or rationalities) and the four behavioural types, it is possible to make a further connection and see how the one maps onto the other. Individualists, by their nature, find the view that nature is benign the most hospitable, and so the two tend to go hand-in-hand, as in Figure 13.3. Likewise, egalitarians, who are questioning and concerned, find nature ephemeral to suit their world-view. It provides a *raison d'être* for their perspective. Hierarchists, in turn, like to organize and manage, and this fits the mould of nature

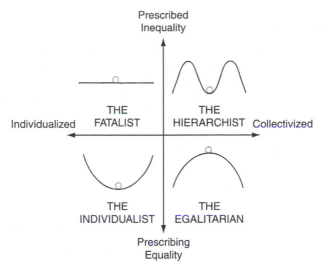

Figure 13.3 The four rationalities

Source: Adams (1995)

which is okay as long as it is properly managed, i.e. perverse/tolerant. This leaves the fatalists, of course, who are presented with the model of nature which is a marble rolling aimlessly on a flat surface. This is the position of those with neither standing nor influence in society, and who feel they are not in control.

Ramifications of cultural theory

The implications of cultural theory, if accepted, are profound. It does not occupy the opposite corner to RAP of Ortwin Renn's classification of theories of risk for nothing (Figure 11.1). RAP is anchored in 'objectivism', the view that risks can be measured, whereas under cultural theory, this has to give way to 'constructivism', the idea that risk is inherently subjective – something that people project onto whatever they observe. This follows because risks are viewed differently, according to which of the four world-views or cultures you subscribe.

Cultural theorists then tell us that because of the fourfold plurality of world-views, it is wrong to impose upon people a decision process framed around one view only (e.g. the hierarchist's RAP), because this disenfranchises all those with other views, and in any case could not win their support since they would see the problem as incorrectly framed. However, they also say that the prospect is not one which rejects science, nor one which accepts extreme forms of relativism, according to which, anyone's opinion is as good as anyone else's (Thompson et al. 1998). In fact, they argue that the fourfold typology is sufficient to encompass much of the diversity of people's views.

Activity 13.3

In order to understand more fully the insights which can be gained from cultural theory, consider the example of global climate change. The following article by John Adams and Michael Thompson (2002) describes how this important challenge for humanity is understood and interpreted by three of the four world-views. As you read the article, reflect upon the following questions:

1 Which world-view is not represented? Why, and does it matter?
2 Which world-view is correct?
3 How should the policy maker react to the different world-views?

 Cultural theory applied to global climate change

An analysis of the global climate change policy debate in the mid-1990s reveals three policy stories. Each policy story provides a setting (the basic assumptions), villains (the policy problem), heroes (policy protagonists), and, of course, a moral (the policy solution). Depending on the socio-institutional context of the particular policy actor, each story emphasized different aspects of the climate change issue.

Profligacy: an egalitarian story

This story begins by pointing to the profligate consumption and production patterns of the North as the fundamental cause of global climate change. Rich industrialized countries, so the argument goes, are recklessly pillaging the world's resources with little regard to the well-being of either the planet or the peoples of its poorer regions. Global climate change is more than an issue that is amenable to quick technical fixes; it is a fundamentally moral and ethical issue.

The setting for this story is a world in which everything is intricately connected with everything else: Nature is Ephemeral. Whether this concerns human society or the natural world, this story urges us to think of Planet Earth as a single living entity. Environmental degradation, then, is also an attack on human well-being. Humans, so the argument goes, have, until now, successfully deluded themselves that they can live apart from the natural environment. In reality, however, there is no place for humans outside nature and thus no particular reason for considering humans as superior to nature. In short, this story is set in an eco-centric world.

The villain in the profligacy story is the fundamentally inequitable structure of advanced industrial society. In particular, the profit motive and the obsession with economic growth – the driving forces of global capitalism – have not only brought us to the brink of eco-logical disaster; they have also distorted our understanding of both the natural and the social world. Global commerce and the advertising industry lead us to desire environ-mentally unsustainable products while our real human needs, living in harmony with nature and with each other, go unfulfilled. What is more, advanced capitalism distributes the spoils of global commerce highly inequitably. This is true within countries (the increasing gap between the rich classes and the poor classes) and among countries (the increasing gap between the affluent countries of the North and the destitute countries of the South). In short, prevailing structural inequalities have led to increasingly unsustainable patterns of consumption and production.

Since everything is connected to everything else, this story continues, we cannot properly understand environmental degradation unless we see it as a symptom of this wider social malaise. The way humans pollute, degrade, and destroy the natural world is merely a very visible indicator for the way they treat each other and particularly the weaker members of society. The logic that allows us to fell thousands of square kilometres of rainforests, to dump toxins in waterways, or pollute the air, is precisely the same logic that produces racism, misogyny, and xenophobia. Tackling one problem inevitably implies tackling all the others.

The heroes of the profligacy story are those organizations and individuals who have managed to see through the chimera of progress in advanced industrial society. They are those groups and persons that understand that the fate of humans is inextricably linked to the fate of Planet Earth. The heroes understand that, in order to halt environmental degradation, we have to address the fundamental global inequities. In short, the heroes of the profligacy policy argument are those organizations of protest such as, most prominently, Greenpeace or Friends of the Earth. These organizations, we need hardly point out, are strongly biased towards the egalitarian social solidarity.

What, then, is the moral of the profligacy story? Its proponents point to a number of solutions. In terms of immediate policy, the profligacy tale urges us to adopt the precautionary principle in all cases: unless policy actors can prove that a particular activity is innocuous to the environment, they should refrain from it. The underlying idea here is that the environment is precariously balanced on the brink of a precipice.

The story further calls for drastic cuts in carbon dioxide emissions; since the industrialized North produces most of these emissions, the onus is on advanced capitalist states to take action. Of course, this policy argument calls for a total and complete ban on chlorofluorocarbons. Yet none of these measures, the story continues, is likely to be fruitful on its own. In order to really tackle the problem of global climate change we in the affluent North will have to fundamentally reform our political institutions and our unsustainable lifestyles. Rather than professionalized democracies and huge centralized administrations, the advocates of the profligacy story suggest we decentralize decision-making down to the grassroots level. Rather than continuing to produce ever-increasing amounts of waste, we should aim at conserving the fragile natural resources we have: we should, in a word, move from the idea of a waste society to the concept of a conserve society. Only then can we meet real human needs. What are real human needs? Simple, they are the needs of Planet Earth.

Population: a hierarchist story

This policy argument tells a story of uncontrolled population growth in the poorer regions of the world. Rapidly increasing population in the South, this story argues, is placing local and global eco-systems under pressures that are fast becoming dangerously uncontrollable: more people means more resource consumption which inevitably leads to environmental degradation. The setting of the population policy story differs slightly, but significantly, from the settings in the other two diagnoses. Like the protagonists of the profligacy story, the population policy argument maintains that global climate change is a moral issue.

Human beings, due to their singular position in the natural world, are the custodians of Planet Earth; since civilization and technological progress have allowed us to understand the natural world more than other species, we have a moral obligation to apply this knowledge wisely. Unlike the profligacy story, the population tale assumes that humans have a special status outside natural processes. The population story, like that of the proponents of the pricing argument (see next story), contends that human actions are rational. However, unlike the pricing argument, the population story tells us the sum of individual rational actions can lead to irrational and detrimental outcomes. The population story, then, is set in a world that needs rational management in order to become sustainable. Yet, while the motive of rational management is an ethical duty to preserve the planet, the means of management are technical. Economic growth, and the socio-economic system that underpins that growth, are necessary components in any global climate change policy response. However, economic growth in itself is no solution: it must be tempered, directed, and balanced by the careful application of knowledge and judgement.

The villain in the population tale is uncontrolled population growth. Since each individual has a fixed set of basic human needs (such as food, shelter, security, etc.) and these needs are then standardized at every level of socio-economic development, population increase, other things being equal, must lead to an increase in the aggregate demand for resources. Humans, the story insists, satisfy their basic human needs by consuming resources. It follows that population growth must lead to an increase in resource consumption: more people will produce more carbon dioxide to satisfy their basic needs. Given the limited nature of most resources, population growth must invariably lead to over-consumption and degradation of natural resources.

The heroes of the population story are those institutions with both the organizational capacities (that is, the technical knowledge) and the 'right' sense of moral responsibility. In short, the global climate change issue should be left to experts situated in large-scale, well-organized administrations. In terms of our typology of organizational types, the population story emerges from hierarchically structured institutions.

The moral of the population story is to rationally control population growth. In particular, this means the introduction of family planning and education in the countries most likely to suffer from rapid population growth. Here, the onus for action is quite clearly on the countries of the South. Rapid population growth has eroded societal management capacities; if we are to tackle the global climate change issue, we must first establish the proper organizational preconditions.

Prices: an individualist story

This story locates the causes of global climate change in the relative prices of natural resources. Historically, prices have poorly reflected the underlying economic scarcities; the result, plain for all to see, is a relative over-consumption of natural resources.

The setting of the prices tale is the world of markets and economic growth. Unlike the profligacy story, the prices diagnosis sees no reason to muddy the conceptual waters with extraneous considerations of social equality. Yes, it says, global climate change is an important issue, but it is an issue that is amenable to precise analytical treatment. It is, in short, a technical issue to which we can apply a technical discourse.

Economic growth, far from being a problem, is the sole source of salvation from environmental degradation. Environmental protection, the proponents of this policy argument contend, is a very costly business. In order, then, to be able to foot the huge bill for adjusting to a more sustainable economy, societies will have to command sufficient funds. These funds, in turn, will not materialize from thin air: only economic growth can provide the necessary resources to tackle the expensive task of greening the economy.

In sum, the prices tale takes place in a world determined by the Invisible Hand (a fundamental premise of classical economists). Here, individuals know and can precisely rank their preferences. In the world of the prices story, individual pursuit of rational self-interest (economic utility) leads, as if by magic, to the optimal allocation of resources. If market forces are allowed to operate as they should, then resource prices will accurately reflect underlying scarcities; the price mechanism then keeps environment-degrading consumption in check. However, if someone (usually the misguided policy maker) meddles with market forces, prices cannot reflect real scarcities; this gives rise to incentives for rational economic actors to over- or under-consume a particular resource.

The villain in the prices story is misguided economic policy. Barriers to international trade, subsidies to inefficient national industries, as well as price and wage floors, introduce distortions to the self-regulatory powers of the market. These distortions have historically led markets to place a monetary value on natural resources that belies the true market value. The result, the protagonists of this policy argument maintain, has been wholesale over-consumption and degradation of the natural world.

The heroes of the prices story are those institutions that understand the economics of resource consumption. In the global climate change debate, these institutions comprise players such as the Global Climate Coalition and trans-national energy companies. In terms of the cultural theory typology, the heroes of this story are those institutions that are strongly permeated by the individualist solidarity.

The moral of the prices story is as simple as its prognosis: in order to successfully face the challenge of global climate change, we have to 'get the prices right'. Unlike the profligacy story, the prices tale sees no necessity to restructure existing institutions. If it is the distortions of global, national and regional market mechanisms that undervalue natural resources, then any climate change policy that fails to remove these distortions is 'fundamentally flawed'. Policy responses must work 'with the market'. Here, concrete policy proposals consist of both general measures, such as the liberalization of global trade, as well as more specific measures, such as carbon taxes or tradable emission permits.

 Feedback

1 You should quickly spot that the fatalists' world-view is absent. This is because fatalists would not be involved in the debate, because they would not expect to be listened to, and their position would be undefined. Whether this matters is a matter of opinion. You could argue that if they have nothing to say or contribute, then why listen? On the other hand, if they can be approached, and convinced that their views will be taken seriously and responded to, then a better policy process will result. Nor should you overlook the fact that even the fatalists can, if strongly motivated by a perceived injustice, take up arms quite effectively.

2 Cultural theorists would argue that if you ask the question, 'Which view is correct?' then you have made a mistake! The three stories tell plausible but conflicting tales of climate change. All three tales use reason and logic to argue their points. None of the tales is 'wrong', in the sense of being implausible or incredible. Yet, at the same time, none of the stories is completely 'right'; each argument focuses on those aspects of climate change for which there is a suitable solution cast within the terms of a particular world-view.

3 To quote Adams and Thompson (2002):

In a policy process where politics matters (that is, in any policy process) there will always be at least three divergent but plausible stories that frame the issue, define the problem, and suggest solutions. Thus conflict in policy-making processes is endemic, inevitable, and desirable, rather than pathological, curable or deviant. Any policy process that does not take this into account does so at the risk of losing political legitimacy.

Therefore, the message for the policy maker is that these voices must all be listened to and accommodated, as far as possible, in the decision process.

Adams (1995) likens it to 'moving up the insight axis' as shown in Figure 13.4. This is where policy makers must try to locate themselves – above the fray so that they can discern and be detached from the competing explanations and concerns, and thus be better placed to take an even-handed approach which inspires mutual trust.

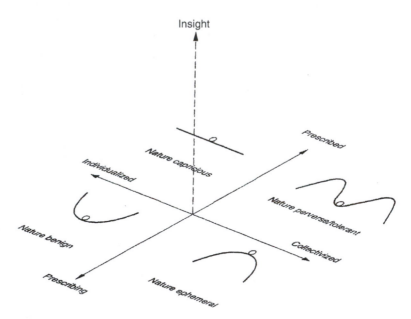

Figure 13.4 The insight axis and 'rising above the fray'
Source: Adams (1995)

Summary

This third model of risk is radically different from those which have gone before. While not at all rejecting the roles for science and economics in policy formulation, it opens up new vistas, demanding that recognition be given to alternative world-views, all of which are seen as legitimate, and each of which points the finger at different causes and different solutions. The task of the policy maker thus now encompasses a powerful need to communicate and listen to stakeholders and anyone affected by policy decisions. The aim of the policy maker must be *to rise above the fray*; to listen, communicate and respond; and to try to accommodate as many concerns as possible into the policy process in the quest for sensible and equitable solutions.

References

Adams J (1995) *Risk*. London: University College London Press.

Adams J and Thompson M (2002) *Taking Account of Societal Concerns about Risk: Framing the Problem*. Sudbury: HSE Books.

Douglas M (1985) *Risk Acceptability According to the Social Sciences*. New York: Russell Sage Foundation.

Rayner S (1992) Cultural theory and risk analysis, in Krimsky S and Golding D (eds) *Social Theories of Risk*. Westport, CT: Praeger.

Schwartz M and Thompson M (1990) *Divided We Stand: Redefining Politics, Technology and Social Choice*. New York: Harvester Wheatsheaf.

Thompson M, Rayner S and Ney S (1998) Risk and governance part II: policy in a complex and plurally perceived world. *Government and Opposition* 33(2): 139–66.

SECTION 5

Other approaches

14 Environmental, social and health impact assessment

Overview

In Section 2 you read about what is nowadays regarded as the classic quantitative method of environmental health risk assessment. However, you are now aware from Section 3 that despite its rapidly expanding global presence, it does not go unchallenged. By no means should this be interpreted as a death knell, for all things, including good things, have their limitations and their detractors. In this section of the book you will read about some alternative approaches to environmental health policy, commencing in this chapter with environmental, social and health impact assessment. This is not at all to say that these alternatives should necessarily usurp the classic method, but that you should be aware of their existence, their merits, and their limitations.

Learning objectives

By the end of this chapter, you will be better able to:

- **describe the processes of environmental, social and health impact assessment**
- **be cognisant of the needs which gave rise to them**
- **compare their strengths and limitations**
- **discuss how they relate to the classical health risk assessment model.**

Key terms

Environmental impact assessment A technique and process by which information about the environmental effects of a project is collected.

Health impact assessment A method which aims to identify the likely changes in health risk of a policy, programme, plan, or development action on a defined population.

Social impact assessment The process of assessing or estimating, in advance, the social consequences that are likely to follow from specific policy actions or project developments.

Strategic environmental assessment The formalized, systematic and comprehensive process of evaluating the environmental effects of a policy, plan or programme and its alternatives.

Sustainability Development which meets the needs of the present without compromising the ability of future generations to meet their own needs.

Tools for environmental policy

The growing interest of the public in the state of the environment has resulted in international initiatives to safeguard the environment and promote sustainability. An early example was the requirement in some countries for environmental impact assessments (EIA) to be carried out on new development projects to ensure that their impacts are taken into account. While it is true that healthy environments and healthy populations are inter-related, it nonetheless came to be felt that EIAs as such did not fully integrate health concerns, which tended to be dealt with through the provision of health care services and discrete public health legislation. For this reason, there have been moves to introduce specific environmental management tools which focus upon health – health impact assessments (HIA) – or to more fully integrate health issues into EIAs (HEIA). For those whose interest is ecosystems, ecological risk assessment is a further approach, though very much in its infancy.

However, just as there exists potential for development projects to give rise to health impacts, benign or malignant, the same must also be true at the policy level. One example is agricultural policy which can have health impacts through food quality, access to food, nutritional status of the affected population, environmental disruption, the supply and nature of jobs, or other implications such as the introduction of new varieties such as rape seed with their allergenic properties (BMA 1998). In fact, health consequences may be associated with all levels of activity, from policies to plans, programmes and projects. This has given rise to a further suite of strategic-level management tools for assessing health impacts, including strategic environmental assessment (SEA), social impact assessment (SIA), and the like. This chapter discusses these initiatives, starting with EIA.

Project environmental impact assessment

Environmental impact assessment is normally applied at the project level. Projects might include things like changing the use of land from forest to agriculture, or the construction of anything from wells, to drainage schemes, dams, roads, factories, and even tourism resorts.

EIA has been defined as follows:

A technique and process by which information about the environmental effects of a project is collected, both by the developer and from other sources, and taken into account by the planning authority in forming their judgements on whether the development should go ahead.

(DoE 1989)

The generic process is outlined in Figure 14.1. You should note in particular that consultation with stakeholders, and their potential participation, is seen as an integral part of the process. This is an issue which will be revisited many times in this book. For the moment, it is useful to be reminded that three main theoretical justifications have been given for increased participation. Academics refer to these reasons as *normative*, *epistemological*, and *instrumental*, grand terms whose meanings are relatively simple – see Table 14.1.

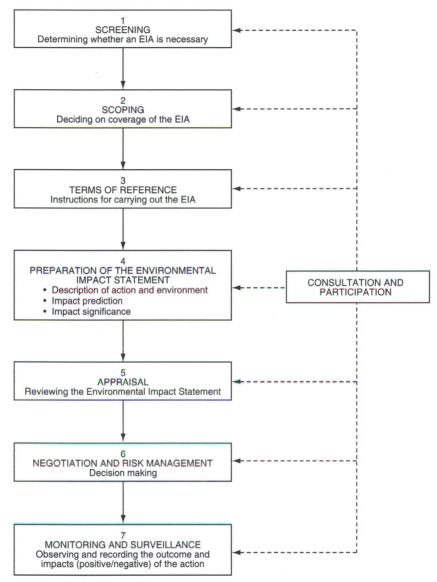

Figure 14.1 A generic EIA process
Source: BMA (1998)

✎ **Activity 14.1**

In contemplating the pervasive role for stakeholder consultation and participation in EIA as proposed in Figure 14.1, make some notes on how this sits with the various models of environmental decision making that you have encountered earlier (e.g. RAP, the psychometric paradigm, and cultural theory).

Table 14.1 The cited advantages of broadening participation in the EIA process

Nature of goal	Description
Normative	Broadening participation is in the interests of democracy because environmental policy decisions are not value-free
Epistemological	Decision makers do not know everything and can benefit from knowledge outside of traditional regulatory structures
Instrumental	Broadening participation helps ensure the political acceptability of resulting policy decisions

Source: Adapted from Rothstein (2004)

 Feedback

A strict RAP model might well not see the need for this consultation. After all, if risks have been properly assessed, if stakeholders are rational actors (individual utility maximizers), and if their values have been properly assessed by WTP techniques, then RAP should incorporate everything they care about, and Pareto optimization will determine the best path. On the other hand, the psychometric paradigm might well say, 'Hold on, the concerns of the stakeholders may be legitimate even if they are not strictly "rational" in RAP's terms. We must elicit their concerns and at least consider factoring them into the decision process.' And, as you might guess, cultural theorists would be appalled at RAP's arrogance, demanding that consultation permeate the entire process.

Many countries now have a legal requirement that new, substantive programmes, such as dam-building, must undertake an EIA; this includes major development projects funded by the World Bank. This is directly related to the declaration at the UN conference on Environment and Development that 'human beings were at the centre of concern for sustainable development' and so development projects now must prepare EIAs.

As shown in Figure 14.1, EIAs will in part follow a similar pattern to quantitative risk assessment, with hazards being identified, dose–response relationships sought, and emissions assessed from the project's technical specifications. To assess exposure and hence impacts, this primary data must be combined with secondary data on population and geography and possibly other factors too. These processes are necessary for every aspect of interest, for example, noise, air quality, or water supply. As this process is supposed to occur prior to the commencement of the project, there is little opportunity for new research and so the assessment has to be based on existing scientific knowledge. In practice this means that data must be extrapolated from other situations and assumptions. As reported by the Ministry of Environment and Forests of India (2006), EIA studies require not only a lot of primary data (such as air and water quality) but also much secondary environmental data on demography, forestry, watersheds, land use, geology and ecology, and this has often been a major bottle neck in achieving the full benefits of EIA.

Activity 14.2

Write down as many elements as you can think of that could be included in an environmental impact assessment. Use a specific local or regional example with which you are familiar. The following categories will help you to structure your answer:

- environmental pollution and ecological considerations
- use of natural resources
- social effects
- economic factors.

 Feedback

Look at Table 14.2 for a comprehensive list of the variety of possible environmental impacts of a development project, and compare it with the items you noted down.

Table 14.2 Examples of environmental impacts or effects

Cause	Effect
Pollution and ecological considerations	Effects on air, water, noise and vibration levels, radiation levels, flora and fauna, ecology, biological diversity, contamination levels, health, areas of outstanding natural beauty, natural and artificial landscapes, historical and cultural heritage, visual environment and aesthetics, traffic generation and management, soil erosion and land degradation, drainage and sewerage, open space, waste generation and management, and climate.
Use of natural resources	Effects on agricultural land, forest resources, water supplies (including groundwater), minerals and marine resources, energy resources, building materials, wetlands, mangroves, coral, rainforest, wilderness and bush.
Social effects	Effects on settlement patterns, employment, land use, housing, social life, welfare, recreational facilities, community facilities and services, accessibility, safety, residential amenity, indigenous communities, minority groups, youth, the unemployed, the aged, the disabled, women, and the socioeconomic profile of the affected community.
Economic factors	Effects on accessibility to facilities, services and employment opportunities, urban infrastructure, choice and affordability of goods and services, the local rate base, infrastructure costs and contributions, real income, land prices and the likely multiplier effect.

What could happen if you don't do an EIA? To understand how environmental impact assessments can make a positive contribution to health, environment and project development, it is instructive to look at a development project carried out before EIAs were required. The following, adapted from WHO/CEMP (1992), describes the Lower Seyhan irrigation project in Turkey, highlighting the positive and negative consequences of the project.

The Lower Seyhan irrigation project in Turkey

In the 1950s a huge irrigation project was started in the Cukurova region. The project included the construction of a dam on the Seyhan River to store water for hydro-electric and agricultural purposes; the establishment of a spillway for excess water; construction of irrigation channels to distribute the water throughout the plain and for the irrigation of fields.

The authorities did not consider it a danger when workers from the south of Turkey arrived with malaria. It was thought that the disease was totally under control because of the very low number of cases reported in the country. The consequences of the project were:

1 Populations from areas to be covered with water were resettled around newly irrigated areas.
2 Productivity of irrigated lands increased.
3 Insects and different kinds of insecticides were introduced to the area, creating vector resistance to insecticides.
4 Irrigation increased the number of arable fields, creating an increase in the need for labourers.
5 People moved from the poorer parts of the country (mostly from areas that still had malaria epidemics) to be seasonal workers in the newly developed areas.
6 Seasonal workers settled along the canals (attracted by the vegetation and the gentle slopes), where water collections became efficient breeding places for malaria vectors.
7 Malaria parasites were introduced to the local mosquito vector (*An sacharovi*) which has a great capacity for transmitting the disease.
8 Industries increased their work on local products because of the agricultural development.
9 The increase in industrial activity created a further demand for workers.
10 Workers and families gravitated towards industrial activities, resulting in an increase in population for the Cukurova region.
11 Unhealthy settlements were established around towns for the incoming populations.
12 New, high rise apartment buildings were built to meet the housing needs of the newcomers. The underground floors of these buildings became new breeding places for vectors because of the high level of the water table and deep basement excavation.
13 Malaria parasites were transmitted to non-immune people.
14 Finally, there was a resurgence of malaria in the area. During 1970, the number of cases reported in the Cukurova region increased from 49 to 149.

 Activity 14.3

If an EIA had been required before the project started, and the significance of malaria-infected workers understood, what could have been done to mitigate the risk?

 Feedback

Malaria-infected workers could have been excluded or treated, and any new cases could have been monitored and treated. New housing in the towns could have been built without the possibility of standing water in the basements. Proper provision would have been made to house seasonal agricultural workers away from the shanty towns on the water's edge, and industrial workers could have been provided with accommodation of an adequate standard.

EIAs have been criticized because there has been a tendency to concentrate on immediate, biophysical consequences of programmes or projects, omitting consideration of social effects of development projects. They have also been criticized for a lack of health expertise, with conclusions being drawn on the basis of comparison with environmental quality criteria (for example, soil, air and water quality standards) rather than fully-fledged health risk assessments. Another perceived shortcoming has been that they are normally applied at the project level, and therefore miss out the cumulative effects of broader initiatives at the policy level. This has given rise to the technique of strategic environmental assessment (SEA).

Strategic environmental assessment (SEA)

The simple definition of SEA is that it is the environmental assessment of any strategic action, whether at the level of policy, plan or programme. More specifically, it has been defined as:

the formalised, systematic and comprehensive process of evaluating the environmental effects of a policy, plan or programme and its alternatives, including the preparation of a written report on the findings of that evaluation, and using the findings in publicly accountable decision-making.

(Thérivel and Partidário 1996)

SEAs differ from EIAs in that they offer a much better opportunity to address the cumulative impacts of many individual projects, any linkages to other policies, and sustainability issues. Despite their strategic nature, SEAs can be applied at every level from national and international, to regional or local.

As an example of a local application, consider the Bara Operational Forest Management Plan (OFMP) of the Kingdom of Nepal (Khadka et al. 1996). The OFMP was believed to be necessary to permit commercialization of timber and fuel wood production in the Bara District forest. It had many apparent advantages, including better management of dwindling forest species, provision of jobs, forest regeneration, and protection of sensitive areas. However, it was clear that the implementation of such a plan would have an array of adverse as well as beneficial impacts associated with the biophysical, social and economic aspects of the area. It was thus important to analyse the plan prior to implementation so that negative consequences could be avoided or minimized cost-effectively. Approximately 150 impacts were identified through stakeholder consultation and these were discussed in a series of workshops open to all. The following edited extracts from an article by Ram Khadka and colleagues provide information on the main issues which were identified by this SEA.

Issues identified in the OFMP SEA

Involvement of local people

About 10 per cent of people in Bara District are poor and landless, and earn their liveli-
hood through exploitation of forest resources. They will be affected by the plan, particularly due to changes in tenure. The employment of such people in the project is necessary
for implementation to be successful. The OFMP prescribes involvement of local people,
but lacks details of how training, education and awareness raising will be undertaken; it has
no budget for this either.

Uncontrolled forest burning

Forest burning is used to clear land for farming and settlement. The significance of this
impact is high, since the fire kills regenerating saplings and often destroys the crowns of
trees. Uncontrolled burning needs to be restricted.

Poaching of timber and fuel wood

Illegal logging and sale of wood are major problems and have led to massive deforestation.
The implementation of the OFMP might reduce such impacts by creating jobs. However,
the current plan does not provide details and cost implications of employing local people.

Poaching of wildlife

Local people supplement their income by illegal capture of wildlife. While implementation
of the OFMP may make poaching more difficult, it offers no solutions, nor does it discuss its
own impact on the area's wildlife habitats.

Domestic fuel wood gathering

Most people in Bara District use the forest as a source of fuel wood for cooking. Implementation of the OFMP would increase supply eventually, but there might be a dislocation
of supply during the early stages. The plan fails to address this.

Clearing the forest for agriculture and settlement

The establishment of the OFMP might stabilize the forest which is being continually pushed
back, but would give rise to short term social disruption which needs to be addressed.

Employment

Although the OFMP would create jobs which currently are non-existent, more work is
needed to quantify the number and for how long. The plan does not indicate if wages are
included.

Grazing of animals

Grazing of livestock is said to prevent forest regeneration. This would be prevented under
the OFMP, but it is not said how it would be implemented nor what the alternatives are for
local people.

Soil erosion

Soil erosion is important in some areas, but these are outside the area covered by the plan.
However, road construction and logging may still affect these areas. Prescriptions are
needed for minimizing soil erosion.

Loss of habitats and biodiversity

This is important politically, because of international perceptions of how Nepal's remaining forests are being managed. The OFMP recognizes this, but needs to create a well-planned biodiversity strategy.

Tenure rights of local people

The plan needs to acknowledge more strongly the issue of tenure and how it will be resolved.

Legal and institutional arrangements

Legislation requires the plan not to affect the environment significantly. The plan needs to show sufficient grounds that this is the case.

Timber harvesting methods

The plan needs to outline how the potential negative impacts of timber harvesting will be avoided. A series of harvesting guidelines would be useful in this respect.

Silvicultural practices

The OFMP describes silvicultural activities but more information is needed on negative impacts and effects on animal and plant habitats.

 Activity 14.4

What was the coverage of the study and what were the implications of its findings for the true nature of the OFMP?

 Feedback

The SEA study was commendable for its comprehensiveness in terms of socio-economic, ecological and political impacts, but, although it did receive some consideration, health impacts are not directly mentioned in this list. Regarding the OFMP, Khadka et al. (1996) actually maintain that this more closely resembles a timber management plan than a forest management plan, and lacks sufficient consideration of biophysical, social and cultural aspects related to forest resource utilization.

Despite criticisms, SEA has many potential benefits as identified by Sadler and Baxter (1997). SEA does the following:

* promotes integrated environment and development decision making;
* facilitates the design of environmentally sustainable policies and plans;
* provides for consideration of a larger range of alternatives than is normally possible in project EIA;
* takes account, where possible, of cumulative effects and global change;
* strengthens and streamlines project EIA by prior identification of impacts and information requirements, clearance of strategic issues and concerns, and reduces time and effort to conduct reviews.

Social impact assessment (SIA)

Project EIAs have generally been formulated with the physical rather than the social environment in mind, with the emphasis on conservation of nature, ecology, and sustainability. Typical considerations include traffic, air pollution and climate. Social impacts are often under-estimated. So apart from the insufficiency of EIA at the strategic level, which SEA attempts to rectify, this further deficit needed to be addressed. This contributed to the emergence of the concept of social impact assessment (SIA).

As a potential example of the utility of SIA, the following edited extract from a New Zealand government website (New Zealand Government 2006) describes concerns over the social impacts of the proposed provision of broadband internet access to rural and urban areas.

 Activity 14.5

As you read it, make notes about the author's attitude to the following:

1 Why policy makers should be cautious in what outwardly appears to be a valid way of extending democracy.
2 The reasons why these arguably important social impacts are often neglected. Add your own thoughts about this too.

 Disadvantages of technology to Māori

Māori continue to feature disproportionately in almost all of the negative statistics including unemployment, education, health, housing, domestic abuse, crime, and of course limited technological capacity.

There is a strong perception of potential negative impacts of increased reliance upon broadband communication on Māori societies including in particular those upon Māori women, tamariki, and high users of Government services such as unemployed and single parents. Informants say there is already a problem where Māori who are behind in their knowledge of Government systems may be disadvantaged further if services are provided online and not face to face. Disadvantages, they say, are exacerbated by a lower level of access to services, improper use of services, and the likelihood of delayed participation.

While some access issues relate to rural Māori, some say there are assumptions that Māori who live in cities have good access to technology and related services such as cyber cafés. However, there are clearly disparities within urban environments. For example, the 2001 NZ Census shows that in some suburbs with a high demographic of Māori and Pacific peoples, access to the Internet and Internet services is poor and correlates with other disparities.

The idea of cultural and social impact in relation to technology is not new and has been the subject of scrutiny for decades. The problem is that it is often discarded as eccentric, minimalised as scaremongering, or is retrospective (after the fact).

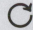

Feedback

1 The author surmises that rather than being an extension of democracy, that the move will exacerbate social inequalities because a practical consequence of the provision of broadband would be a loss of face-to-face contact which is the preferred method of communication by some social groups. It therefore needs to be thought through in more detail.

2 As the author says, although recognition of social and cultural impacts of technology is not new, it is often discarded as eccentric and minimalized. Why should this occur? Social and cultural theorists might well argue that it is in part attributable to the fragmentation of society. Technical decisions about things like broadband are generally delegated to technical people whose strength is seldom in the social implications of their technologies.

In the following extract, Susan Joyce (2001), a Canadian researcher, notes that attitudes to the *desirability* of SIA also extend to the *meaning* of SIA. In this account, Joyce refers to a 'technocratic approach' which is clearly a reference to what we have previously described as RAP.

The technocratic approach and the participatory approach

The technocratic approach regards SIA as a rational mechanism for assessing impacts. The task of the SIA practitioner is seen to be one of providing reasoned and dispassionate information to centralized decision-makers that operate in an environment in which politics are subordinated to technical analysis.

At the other extreme, the participatory approach to SIA has evolved from a desire to incorporate the actor's perspectives into SIA. This approach views society and social goals as pluralistic and conflicting. Social reality is seen to be subjective, bounded and defined by social rules and meanings formed by the actors within it. The subjective perspective of all stakeholders is therefore regarded as intrinsic to the SIA process. As such, the SIA practitioner is seen as the facilitator rather than the arbitrator of knowledge, with the expertise located in the affected culture. With this prioritization given to subjective perspectives, the decision-making process in which SIA is situated is portrayed as value laden and political in character, with the ultimate determinant of action being a value choice.

You will note that this extract is strongly reminiscent of the clash between RAP and alternative social theories, as examined in Chapter 11. The technocratic approach referred to is clearly anchored in RAP, whereas the so-called participatory approach sits astride the opposite corner of Ortwin Renn's classification of social theories of risk (see Figure 11.1).

Joyce herself sees these as *extreme approaches* and proposes that to build on their respective strengths an integrative approach to SIA is needed in which both community and expert opinion contribute to the criteria of significance and acceptability that underpin the impact assessment process. The following edited extract from Joyce (2001) describes two case study reports in which SIA was, allegedly, a success and which Joyce sees as the strongest endorsement for this integrative approach.

Activity 14.6

In reading the extracts, note and comment on the following:
1   the role being assigned to technical experts and the method of evaluating project proposals;
2   the way in which the successfulness of SIA was diagnosed.

 The integrative approach

It is significant to note that the two most frequently cited cases in which SIA dramatically affected project development involved integrative SIAs. The first involved the Berger Inquiry into the likely impacts of a proposed gas pipeline through the Mackenzie Valley (from the western Arctic to Alberta) on the environment and the native communities of the region and its subsequent rejection of the application. The Inquiry used expert testimony and technocratic methods, while simultaneously representing the perspectives of native peoples using consultative processes: he went out and listened to the communities. The implication for the Inquiry, and SIA, was that the proposed pipeline project had to be evaluated not according to technical or value-free criteria, but rather in terms of the vision of the people whose communities it would affect. Where the technical model of SIA focused on economic well-being as measured by income and employment, the political model emphasized social well-being, self-determination, and the centrality of cultural values and social institutions.

The second case concerns an SIA of a proposed mine at Coronation Hill in the Northern Territories of Australia. Again, the SIA involved an integrative approach, 'designed to overcome many of the conceptual and methodological flaws observed in more traditional approaches'. According to Ross [quoted by Joyce] the approach recognized that:

> In predicting the potential impacts of forthcoming developments or policies, the people's own predictions, in the form of optimism and fears, are a significant component of people's behaviour and hence of the impacts. This does not diminish the role of the experts or other informed outsiders in making analyses that a community might otherwise be unaware of, contributing technical knowledge and experience beyond that already possessed by the community.

In the SIA, it was concluded that the effect of mining at Coronation Hill would be too adverse for the Jawoyn Aborigines, especially those traditionally affiliated with the spiritual site at Coronation Hill. As a result, Australia's federal cabinet voted against the development.

 Feedback

1   The role of technical experts is still regarded as essential though not as dominant as once it might have been. This shift is reflected in the perceived nature of the assessment criteria used for project evaluation, which were seen to be socio-political rather than technical.

2 There is some inference that the success of SIA was measured by the outcomes of the inquiries, namely that both projects failed to win approval. However, this is not strictly proven because it may be that, for example, the economic cases were weak. Only history can tell if the decisions were actually for the best and even then, it might, as discussed by Eiser (p 154), be imponderable.

Health impact assessment

The spur for the development of HIA has been a perception that while human health has often been taken into account in EIAs and SEAs, assessments tend to estimate only the negative effects resulting from expected changes in (physical) environmental media, neglecting the effects of modifications on other health determinants, such as socio-economic ones, and the possibility of promoting health benefits (UNECE 2004). The effective management of health and other environmental risks also requires medical input, often lacking in traditional EIAs. This requirement arises because of the complexity of health impacts attributable to synergistic effects of different hazards, cumulative effects of chronic exposures, and the differing vulnerabilities of members of the community to adverse effects.

The British Medical Association (1998) says that the failure to fully integrate, or even give attention to, the relationships between the biophysical environment and human health remains a major deficiency in a number of countries, including the UK, and proposes as a solution an approach which overtly integrates HIA into EIA. Figure 14.2 shows how the EIA process (as in Figure 14.1) could be adapted. During scoping and screening the point is made that all five main categories of health detriment should be specifically considered. These are described by the BMA as follows:

- *communicable disease*, e.g. sexually transmitted diseases, infections, micro-biological food contamination;
- *non-communicable disease*, e.g. chronic poisoning, lung disease associated with dust, noise, vibration;
- *inappropriate nutrition*, e.g. deprivation, access to food, pesticide or other chemical contamination;
- *injury*, e.g. traffic injury, violence, occupational injury;
- *mental disorder*, e.g. stress, chronic depression, substance abuse.

By doing this, a medical model is imposed upon the process. Further, rather than attempt to quantify risks associated with identified hazards, which the BMA regards as a difficult and distant goal whose validity is further brought into question because people perceive risks differently, they recommend a simple ranking procedure as more realistic. This might take the form of identifying, for each of the health hazards associated with the activity, the health change as a result of carrying it out. This, the BMA proposes, might be done simply, for example, in terms of: no apparent change, increased risk, or decreased risk. Table 14.3 is suggested as one way of presenting such data.

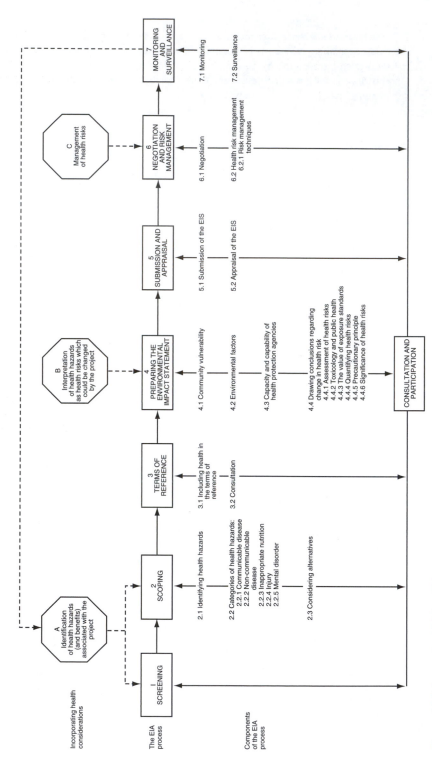

Figure 14.2 Integrating HIA into EIA

Source: BMA (1998)

Health impact assessment for a public water supply project

You have been asked to carry out a health impact assessment as part of a feasibility study for the provision of water standpipes in each street in a poor urban area. The previous water supply came from contaminated wells which were some distance from the main dwelling locations. Communicable diseases have already been identified as the main health issue in this area, but the other forms of health impact should not be discounted.

 Activity 14.7

Use Table 14.3 to record the potential health impacts of the new proposal. State whether they are positive or negative impacts, and make a note of your recommendations to the planning committee on whether or not the development should go ahead.

Table 14.3 Health impact assessment of a development project

Health hazard	Examples	Community vulnerability	Environmental factors giving rise to exposure	Capacity and capability to protect health	Changes in health risks attributable to the project
communicable disease					
non-communicable disease					
injury					
malnutrition					
mental disorder					

Source: BMA (1998)

 Feedback

Table 14.4 lists some responses. You might have recommended the provision of adequate drainage for the standpipes to prevent vector breeding conditions in stagnant water. Overall, the positive health benefits seemingly outweigh the negative impacts, providing straightforward safeguards are put in place, so it could be that you would recommend that the development should go ahead provided there are no other anticipated adverse effects.

Table 14.4 Health impact assessment of standpipe provision

Health hazard	Examples	Community vulnerability	Environmental factors giving rise to exposure	Capacity and capability to protect health	Changes in health risks attributable to the project
communicable disease	diarrhoea	all those in community particularly children playing in the street	better water availability curtails spread of diarrhoeal disease in the home	hygiene education should be provided when standpipes are introduced; decreased use of health services	health improvements generally; less diarrhoea with increased water availability for hand washing and preparation of food
non-communicable disease	malaria	community susceptibility is high	pools near standpipes may provide breeding ground for vectors – high transmission potential	poor provision of local health services	remedial measures needed to combat the new hazard
malnutrition					water available for preparation of food, so more time for procurement and cooking
injury	back injury	water carriers		less distance to travel reduces need to carry heavy loads	reduced risk of injury
mental disorder	stress	water carriers		easy availability of clean water allows time for other activities	reduced risk of stress

Summary

Local, regional, national and international concerns for the environment have led to the generation of a range of techniques for assessing the environmental impacts of developments. Initially the focus was on the environmental impact of projects. This gradually expanded to the policy level via the use of strategic-level assessments. More recently there have been moves to include health, socio-economic and political dimensions. In one sense, these trends may be a reflection of acknowledged deficiencies of strict RAP approaches. Also, the issue of sustainability is firmly on the agenda, and this requires a new perspective, one which links grassroots actions with a 'grand plan'. The techniques themselves have their own shortcomings, and this is unsurprising given that some are novel. A noticeable feature is that all, though some more than others, shift the emphasis towards consultative processes and stakeholder engagement and away from what some see as technocratic decision making. Evidence that this works, in terms of improved societal decision making, is awaited.

References

British Medical Association (1998) *Health and Environmental Impact Assessment*. London: Earthscan.

Department of the Environment (1989) *Environmental Assessment: A Guide to the Procedures*. London: HMSO.

Joyce SA (2001) *Social Impact Assessment in the Mining Industry: Current Situation and Future Directions*. Report No. 46. London: International Institute for Environment and Development and World Business Council for Sustainable Development.

Khadka R, McEachern J, Rautiainen O and Uttam SS (1996) SEA of the Bara Forest Management Plan, *Nepal*, in Thérivel R and Partidário MR (eds) *The Practice of Strategic Environmental Assessment*. London: Earthscan.

Ministry of Environment and Forests of India (2006) http://www.eicinformation.org/

New Zealand Government (2006) http://www.e.govt.nz/archive/services/authentication/tikanga-200408/chapter8.html

Rothstein HF (2004) Precautionary bans or sacrificial lambs? Participative risk regulation and the reform of the UK food safety regime. *Public Administration* 82(4): 857–81.

Sadler B and Baxter M (1997) Taking stock of SEA. *Environmental Assessment* 5: 14–16.

Thérivel R and Partidário MR (1996) *The Practice of Strategic Environmental Assessment*. London: Earthscan.

UN Economic Commission for Europe (2004) Human health in the EIA convention and SEA protocol, in *Proceedings of the Espoo Convention on Transboundary Environmental Impact Assessment*. http://www.unece.org/env/eia/health.html

WHO/CEMP (1992) *Environmental and Health Impact Assessment of Development Projects: A Handbook for Practitioners*. London: Elsevier Applied Science.

Environmental risk ranking

Overview

One of the major objections levelled at the traditional approaches to environmental health decision making, based on RAP-style procedures, is that they either only consider criteria that can be monetized, thereby ignoring other things that are important, or that they try to assign monetary values to these 'other things' in questionable ways, in both cases so that standard mathematical optimization procedures can then be deployed, which themselves are challenged. In an attempt to deal with these criticisms, a surprisingly large number of techniques have been devised whose aim is to bring about more holistic rankings and which in some cases avoid the issue of monetization, initially at least. These often go by the name of multi-criteria or multi-attribute techniques, though there are many variants to the nomenclature which can be confusing. In this chapter you will learn about the basics of some of these techniques. Apart from dealing with these objections, you should note that familiarity with these procedures is important for environmental health policy makers, for how else might it be possible to go about the business of assigning priorities?

Learning objectives

By the end of this chapter, you will be better able to:

- **discuss techniques which have been developed to prioritize environmental health hazards**
- **be familiar with the stages of multi-criteria ranking techniques**
- **recognize the potential benefits and limitations of the techniques**
- **understand the nature of remaining controversies.**

Key term

Human exposure – rodent potency index (HERP) An index devised for ranking the risk of potential human carcinogens based on average human exposure and rodent toxicity data.

The ranking of environmental health risks

In this short account it is impossible to explore in detail risk ranking techniques, so the aim is to provide examples demonstrating broad principles. In fact, you have already encountered some forms of risk ranking, or risk prioritization, in earlier chapters. Figure 7.1 (the two-dimensional risk matrix), Figure 10.1 (another version of the matrix), and Table 2.1 (based on the work of Tammy Tengs and colleagues), all have something to offer in terms of prioritization. If you think about it, Figure 12.5 (Paul Slovic's factor analysis) also provides a ranking of many hazards, albeit from a very different perspective.

 Activity 15.1

To consolidate what we have learned, describe and distinguish between the ranking methods in Figure 7.1 and Figures 10.1 and 12.5.

 Feedback

Figure 7.1 provides either a semi-quantitative or qualitative ranking based on the probability of risks and their consequences, and is usually based on expert knowledge. Figure 10.1 goes one step further by thinking also about the cost-effectiveness of potential risk reduction measures. Figure 12.5 is very different, producing a ranking based on the quantified public perceptions of risks which are encapsulated in dimensions of 'dread' and 'familiarity'. Those in the top-right quadrant are potentially 'prioritized' for action.

A method of 'hazard ranking' chemicals

In 1987, Bruce Ames and colleagues devised a technical method of ranking the scale of possible human hazard associated with a wide range of chemical carcinogens to which people are exposed via diet or workplace. A sample of their calculations is shown in Table 15.1. This method is based on working out the ratio (expressed as a percentage) of the average daily human intake, expressed in mg/kg, divided by TD_{50} which is the daily dose rate (in mg/kg) which halves the percentage of tumour-free animals by the end of a standard lifetime. Thus, the higher the number in the left-hand column of Table 15.1, the higher the possible health hazard.

 Activity 15.2

The HERP hazard factors for alcoholic drinks and DDT exposure have been omitted from Table 15.1. Work out what they should be using the data in Table 15.1.

Table 15.1 Ranking possible human cancer hazards with the HERP index

Possible hazard HERP %	Average daily human exposure (USA)	Human dose of rodent carcinogen per person (70 kg) per day	Potency of carcinogen TD_{50} mg/kg/day	
			Rats	Mice
0.00008	PCBs (1984–86)	PCBs 98 ng	1.74	(9.58)
0.0008	Tap water 1 litre (1987–92)	Chloroform 51 µg	(262)	90.3
0.001	Bacon 19 g	Diethylnitrosamine 19 ng	0.0266	(+)
***	DDT (pre-1972 ban)	DDT 13.8 µg	(84.7)	12.8
0.003	Home air (14h/day)	Benzene 155 µg	(169)	77.5
***	Alcoholic beverages, all kinds	Ethyl alcohol 22.8 ml	9110	(—)
6.1	Tetrachloroethylene (dry cleaners 1980–90)	Tetrachloroethylene 433 mg	101	(126)
140	High exposure EDB workers (pre-1977)	Ethylene dibromide 150 mg	1.52	(7.45)

Source: Ames et al. (1987) with updates from Gold et al. (2003). See Gold et al. (2002) for full text.

Note: Parentheses indicate TD_{50} not used in calculation, this being data for the species with the less potent TD_{50}. (−) = negative in cancer test(s); (+) = positive cancer test(s) but not suitable for calculating TD_{50}.

 Feedback

For alcoholic drinks, taking as an approximation the density of alcohol to be equal to 1.0 and noting that 1ml weighs 1g, the calculation is as follows:

$$HERP (\%) = (22,800/70) \div (9,110) \times 100\% = 3.6\%$$

For DDT:

$$HERP (\%) = (13.8 \times 10^{-3}/70) \div (12.8) \times 100\% = 0.002\% \text{ (after rounding)}$$

Some early comparative risk projects

In 1987, concerns were expressed in the USA about whether the Environmental Protection Agency (EPA) was making the best use of its resources, that is, 'were its activities properly prioritised with the most serious hazards receiving the greatest attention?' As a consequence, the National Comparative Risk Project was instigated, the aim of which was to assess 30 hazards for which EPA had responsibilities (Table 15.2) against four risk criteria (US EPA, 1987). The risk criteria were: human cancer risk, human non-cancer risk, ecological risk, and welfare risk. Each hazard was assessed and ranked against each criterion, but a combined ranking was not attempted. Despite a number of recognized limitations, the study was sufficient to show that there was a mismatch between rankings by experts and those reflected in public opinion.

Table 15.2 The EPA's 1987 list of environmental issues for ranking

1	Primary air pollutants (sulphur dioxide, ozone, etc.)
2	Hazardous/ toxic air pollutants
3	Other air pollutants
4	Radon gas (indoors)
5	Other indoor air pollution
6	Radiation
7	Substances suspected of depleting stratospheric ozone
8	Carbon dioxide
9	Direct point-source discharges to surface waters
10	Indirect point-source discharges to surface waters
11	Non-point source discharges to surface waters
12	Contaminated sludge
13	Discharges to estuaries and oceans
14	Drinking water supplies
15	Active hazardous waste sites
16	Inactive waste sites
17	Municipal waste sites
18	Industrial waste sites
19	Mine wastes
20	Accidental releases of toxics
21	Accidental oil spills
22	Leaks from storage tanks
23	Other groundwater contamination
24	Pesticide residues on food
25	Pesticide application
26	Other pesticide risks
27	New toxic chemicals
28	Biotechnology
29	Consumer product exposure
30	Occupational exposure to chemicals

The matter was revisited, in more detail, by the US Strategic Advisory Board (SAB). The SAB set up three committees – on ecology and welfare, human health, and strategic options – to take the work forward. The committees were comprised of scientists, engineers and environmental managers. The ecology and welfare committee assessed and rated the hazards, including some new ones, against the following criteria: spatial extent of problem, importance of affected ecosystem,

Table 15.3 Summary of SAB's ecological risk ranking work
Key: HHH > HH > H > M > L where HHH = highest etc.

Hazard	Extent of stress			Medium			Recovery time		
	Biosphere	Regional	Ecosystem	Air	Water	Land	Short	Medium	Long
Global climate	HHH	HHH	HHH	HHH					X
Habitat alteration	HH	HHH	HHH		HHH	HHH		X	X
Stratospheric ozone	HHH	HHH	HHH	HHH					X
Biological depletion		HH	HHH		HH	HHH			X
Biocides		M	HH	HH	HH			X	
Toxics in surface waters		M	HH		HH			X	
Acid deposition		H	H	H				X	
Airborne toxics	M	HH	HH	HH				X	
Nutrient release			H		H		X		
Biological oxygen demand			M		M		X		
Turbidity			M		M		X		
Oil			M		M	L	X		
Groundwater		L	L		L				
Radionuclides		L	L	L	L			X	X
Acid inputs to surface waters			H		H			X	
Thermal pollution			L		L		X		

Source: SAB (1990)

potential to cause ecological effects, intensity of exposure and potential for recovery. Table 15.3 shows the ratings achieved and how they were expressed. Note that the hazards are rated in terms of their harmfulness and not their potential for amelioration.

The human health committee identified primary air pollutants, hazardous air pollutants, indoor radon, indoor air pollution excluding radon, drinking water pollutants, pesticide application and occupational chemical exposure as deserving high rank. However, they were cautious about developing an aggregate ranking of agents because the attributable health effects were so disparate.

Activity 15.2

Read the following passage by SAB and note the nature of the problem they experienced. Can you suggest ways by which SAB's problem could be overcome?

Comparing harms

. . . to attempt a relative ranking in terms of severity of such disparate health outcomes as birth defects in infants compared to paralysis in older persons, requires consideration of many dimensions of the values we place on various members of society, families and the utility of specific physical and mental functions for individuals and society. Such a comparison requires that the impact of each effect be scored for severity, a process necessitating selection of suitable measures and scales of severity, as well as appropriate weighting factors. In addition, the current disparity in risk assessment approaches for carcinogens and systemic toxicants makes it exceedingly difficult to construct a universally acceptable aggregate ranking.

Feedback

There is a major difficulty in comparing health detriments (harms) of different kinds. You touched on issues of this kind in Chapter 9 when radiological harms were being considered. There are many dimensions of harm which would need to be considered, including severity of pain, duration of harm, loss of life-years, loss of ability to function, and so on. A great deal of work has now been done on establishing multi-dimensional scales for comparing health states, however. These include scales which go by the name of QALY (quality-adjusted life years), and DALY (disability adjusted life year).

From the perspective of environmental health policy, it is instructive to consider the criteria devised by SAB's Strategic Options Committee for the purpose of evaluating the risk reduction options for dealing with the various hazards.

Activity 15.3

Before reading the SAB Committee's list of eight criteria, try drawing up your own list of criteria for evaluating risk reduction interventions. It might help to think of a few examples of interventions and work from there.

Feedback

The eight criteria are shown in Table 15.4. Note that cost is considered from two perspectives – that of the EPA itself, and that of society. Dependability, or certainty, is another key factor along with implementability. And, as you would expect, the amount of risk reduction which the measure is expected to achieve is listed. There is little point in investing in measures which provide little benefit in terms of risk reduction. In fact, SAB elected to look at this through the fractional, or relative, change in risk, and that resulted in a nationwide discussion about the use of risk-based measures as a means of setting priorities. Table 15.4 also includes cost-effectiveness. There is no mention of cost–benefit, but it is inescapable that this would not surface, explicitly or implicitly, when the viability of control options was debated.

Table 15.4 SAB's assessment criteria for risk reduction options

Annual cost to EPA of implementing the strategy

Cost to society (public and private) of the strategy

Dependability (degree of assurance that the strategy will achieve desired risk reduction)

Speed of risk reduction following implementation of strategy

Implementability and enforceability

Risk reduction (the fraction by which the existing risk would be reduced)

Cost-effectiveness

Short-term and long-term desirability of the strategy

Source: SAB (1990)

Comparative risk assessment

The EPA's pioneering work was aptly entitled 'Unfinished business'. Since that time, a number of agencies, regional authorities and communities around the world have sought to prioritize their activities just as EPA set out to do (Clarence-Davies 1996; HSE 1997). All systems for ranking or prioritizing need to be purpose-designed for the institutional and cultural setting at hand, but certain characteristics, and issues, can be expected to occur often. The general procedure is in fact to carry out the following sequence of steps (Morgan et al. 1995):

1   List the risks to be ranked (prioritized).
2   Identify the risk attributes (characteristics) to be considered.
3   Describe the risks in terms of the attributes.
4   Decide who is going to do the ranking.
5   Perform the rankings and combine the rankings for the different attributes.
6   Summarize the results.

Table 15.2 is one example of a Stage 1 output, albeit for a large agency with a very broad remit. Ranking exercises need not be as demanding as this. Stage 2 is about the assessment criteria (attributes/characteristics). An important issue here is who should identify the criteria. If left to technical experts, there will be, as you have seen in Chapter 12, a tendency to focus on fatality rates and possibly little else, but if the aim is to engage the wider community, other criteria too may be appropriate. Also, what is included depends on the aim of the ranking process. For example, consider Table 15.5 which originates from the government of the State of Vermont (1991) and which aimed to answer the question: 'What environmental problems pose the most serious risks to Vermont and Vermonters?'

Table 15.5 Vermont's quality of life criteria

Criterion	Examples of negative impacts
Aesthetics	Reduced visibility Noise, odours, dust, water weeds, turbidity, grime on buildings Visual impacts from degradation of natural or agricultural land
Economic well-being	Higher cost of fixing, replacing, or buying items or services Lower income or higher taxes due to the problem Loss of jobs as a result of the problem Health care costs and lost productivity
Fairness	Unequal distribution of costs and benefits
Future generations	Shifting the costs of today's activities to those not yet born
Peace of mind	Feeling threatened by possible hazards in the air or water, or by potentially risky facilities
Recreation	Loss of access to recreation lands Degraded quality of recreation land
Sense of community	Rapid growth in population or number of structures in towns Loss of mutual respect Individual liberty exercised at expense of common good Loss of connection between people and the land

Source: Vermont Agency of Natural Resources (1991)

The criteria listed are known as 'Vermont's quality of life criteria', and are a consolidation of what the people of Vermont said were important to them. Alternatively, Table 15.6 shows a much simpler, four-dimensional, ranking system which was devised by Granger Morgan and colleagues (1995) for use by government agencies.

Table 15.6 Suggested format of a risk summary sheet

Criterion	Assessment parameter	How expressed
Number of people affected	Annual expected fatalities	Annual number of person-years lost (range and central estimate)
Degree of environmental impact	Area of ecosystem affected by stress or change	Magnitude of environmental impact – modest, etc.
Knowledge	Degree to which impacts are delayed	Quality of scientific understanding – medium etc.
Dread	Catastrophic potential	Outcome equity – medium etc.

Source: Morgan et al. (1995)

Activity 15.4

Comment on the attributes listed in Tables 15.5 and 15.6. In particular, how do they seek to accommodate public and expert concerns?

 Feedback

The Vermont attributes were provided by the public in consultations. One feature of interest is that health risks are not listed as a top level criterion although they are included through 'peace of mind' and 'economic well-being', which are both linked with the overall health of the population. There is a considerable emphasis on economic factors, and on equity in the form of the distribution of costs and benefits in the current generation and between it and future generations. The criteria in Table 15.6 were clearly designed with something quite different in mind. They were in fact devised by decision experts and their content suggests they are aimed at building a bridge between health and environmental experts, who would mainly be concerned about threats to life (and ecology), and public opinion which, as Slovic's work shows, is influenced by qualitative factors summarized in Table 15.6 as 'knowledge' and 'dread'.

Having agreed upon the assessment criteria, Stages 3 to 5 of the process require each of the risks to be rated against each of the assessment criteria. This requires, first, a scale, qualitative or quantitative, to have been devised for each criterion. It also needs to be decided who will do the rating. Normally, though, this stage is seen as a task requiring expertise of some kind: health, ecological, economic, ethics, etc. Stage 5 also refers to combining the scores across the criteria. To do this, it is necessary to decide upon weighting factors for the criteria, unless all have equal weight, which is unlikely. This is a value-laden task and it may be felt appropriate to engage the affected community in this task if not to place it entirely within their jurisdiction. The method for computing the final score, and hence ranking, for each risk can be accomplished by a variety of means. A simple and commonly used approach is to use the following formula:

Combined score for a hazard = (score on attribute A × weighting factor for A)
+ (score on B × weighting for B) +. . . .

for as many attributes as are described. Though the process appears outwardly simple, it has many subtleties and needs care and thought in its application (Keeney and Raiffa 1976; Kiker et al. 2005; DTLGR 2001).

Comparative risk assessment: moral choices

At the beginning of this chapter the idea was advanced that environmental risk ranking might overcome or avoid some of the objections which have been associated with the other approaches to decision making and prioritization described earlier. The abridged passage that follows, by US attorney Frederick Anderson (1996), gives reasons why the process of comparative risk assessment is viewed as necessary and why nonetheless it still encounters resistance.

Activity 15.5

While reading, focus on and think about:

1 the arguments for and against comparative risk assessment (referred to as 'comparative risk analysis' in this passage);
2 whether comparative risk assessment truly represents an advance or is merely a revamping of the status quo;
3 by what means benefits of comparative risk assessment might be realized.

 Comparative risk analysis

The most frequently advanced justification for comparative risk analysis is economic. We currently spend such huge sums on reducing risks that we cannot afford to do so inefficiently. But there are strong moral grounds for comparative risk analysis. We owe it to ourselves to confront our choices honestly.

It is just this moral dimension which accounts, paradoxically, for a final source of resistance to use of comparative risk analysis. Comparative risk analysis rubs our noses in the choices we must make to solve one problem while neglecting another, or to protect one group while turning away from helping another. Comparative risk analysis asks us to make explicit our implicit choices. We do not want to hear that scarcity is not just an economic law but is part of the human condition, that it can be avoided for some but not for all. When forced to gaze on our choices (as comparative risk analysis makes us do), we want to avert our eyes, to avoid facing the moral consequences of the implicit and explicit decisions made. Yet we have a moral obligation to confront the fact that our implicit choices to protect or leave unprotected, to spend or not to spend, and to allocate scarce resources to less productive uses have consequences just as explicit choices do. Comparative risk analysis, by definition, calls on us to face up to the moral implications of these choices . . .

. . . risk-based priority setting and risk assessment are under attack by environmental advocates who favor legislative strategies based on chemical bans and toxics use reduction. Environmentalists also resist ceding their strong influence on the environmental agenda to priority setting by agencies and scientific organizations . . . Some groups fear comparative risk analysis and risk assessment because they do not understand the quantitative methods employed, do not trust the results presented, and feel excluded from the process that produced the risk assessment ranking. Objections to risk assessment and comparative risk analysis based on data needs, technical content, and delays seem to follow from a prejudgment that a need to regulate exists.

 Feedback

1 The argument for comparative risk analysis is, as with benefit–cost analysis, that it forces you to be honest about resource utilization and the implicit trade-offs. The arguments against are not new either. If your motivation is to ban something outright, or to be a scientific sceptic, then comparative risk analysis, which furthers compromises, is not for you. Furthermore, if you concede that risk analysis has something to offer, then the balance of power might shift away from environmentalism and towards science.

2 Is comparative risk analysis something new, or just something old in fresh clothes? The answer is probably that it depends. It is clear that the technique can take on board other dimensions that people care about, but, like all 'sophisticated' tools, it needs to be handled skilfully and with care. It could either assist decision making, including making it better both technically and more democratic, or it could hinder it.

3 Steps to help realize this dream would include: the use of credible, neutral science in comparative risk assessment; carrying out the process transparently; involving affected parties early; and trying to build consensus.

Summary

Environmental health policy makers ultimately cannot avoid questions of prioritization. These are both difficult and ethically challenging. There is continuing controversy over the relative contributions of science, economics and politics in the process of prioritization. As well as strictly science-based schemes (such as the HERP index), a number of multi-criteria techniques have been devised which attempt to build a bridge by incorporating wider public concerns into the decision process. By and large, these are still at the experimental stage, but despite having their detractors, offer some possibility of a new era in policy making.

References

Ames BN, Magaw R and Swinsky Gold L (1987) Ranking possible carcinogenic hazards. *Science* 236: 271–80.

Anderson FR (1996) CRA and its stakeholders: advice to the Executive Office, in Clarence-Davies J *Comparing Environmental Risks: Tools for Setting Government Priorities*. Washington, DC: Resources for the Future.

Clarence-Davies J (1996) *Comparing Environmental Risks: Tools for Setting Government Priorities*. Washington, DC: Resources for the Future.

Department for Transport, Local Government and the Regions (2001) *Multi-Criteria Analysis: A Manual*. London: DfTLGR.

Gold LS, Slone TH, Manley NB and Ames BN (2003) *Misconceptions about the causes of cancer*. Vancouver: The Fraser Institute.

Health and Safety Executive (1997) *Risk Ranking*. Report No. 131/1997. Sudbury: HSE Books.

HM Treasury (2005) *Managing Risks to the Public: Appraisal Guidance*. London: HM Treasury.

Keeney RL and Raiffa H (1976) *Decisions with Multiple Objectives: Preferences and Value Trade-Offs*. Cambridge: Cambridge University Press.

Kiker GA, Bridges TS, Varghese A, Seager TP and Linkov I (2005) Application of multicriteria decision analysis in environmental decision making. *Integrated environmental Assessment and Management* 1(2): 95–108.

Morgan MG, Fischhoff B, Lave L and Fischbeck P (1995) A proposal for ranking risk within federal agencies, in: Clarence-Davies J *Comparing Environmental Risks: Tools for Setting Government Priorities*. Washington, DC: Resources for the Future.

Strategic Advisory Board (1990) *Reducing Risk: Setting Priorities and Strategies for Environmental Risk*. Report No. EPA-SAB-EC-90-021. Washington, DC: US EPA.

US EPA (1987) *Unfinished Business: A Comparative Assessment of Environmental Problems*. Washington, DC: US EPA.

Vermont Agency of Natural Resources (1991) *Environment 1991: Risks to Vermont and Vermonters*. Waterbury, Vermont: VANR.

Overview

In the previous two chapters you have read about a number of alternatives, or supplements, to risk assessment. In this chapter you will review another approach, known as alternatives assessment, and consider how it stands in relation to those already considered. You will also explore the nature and significance of the frequently cited 'precautionary principle'.

Learning objectives

By the end of this chapter, you will be better able to:

- **outline the process of alternatives assessment**
- **locate environmental health risk assessment in a broader framework of aids for policy analysis**
- **understand how the idea of precaution and the precautionary principle link up with what you have learnt about environmental health policy making.**

Key term

Alternatives assessment A process that involves looking at the risks, benefits and other pros and cons of a broad range of environmental health policy options.

Criticizing 'risk ranking'

Environmental risk ranking and comparative risk assessment are, as you saw in Chapter 15, new initiatives aimed at helping society prioritize environmental actions while taking on board broader concerns than those normally considered by conventional risk assessment and cost–benefit analysis. But do they go far enough?

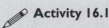 **Activity 16.1**

The following passage by Mary O'Brien (2000), consultant on alternatives to risk assessment, criticizes the sufficiency of these initiatives. In reading the passage, think about these questions:

1   What is the nature of her argument?
2   Can you think of examples in support of her case?
3   Why might these arguments be resisted?

 Environmentally responsible behaviour

If we have a goal of preventing and solving environmental problems, rather than choosing which ones to ignore, we will not ask which types of environmental degradation are worst. Instead, we will ask 'how do we get industry, the government, and citizens to behave more carefully toward the environment?' This question focuses on conditions that encourage or require environmentally responsible behaviours.

It is noteworthy that comparative risk assessment processes rank environmental problems. It would be just as logical to rank which behaviours are causing the greatest environmental problems, or who is causing the greatest environmental problems, or which social arrangements allow or encourage people to cause environmental problems. By focusing on environmental problems rather than on problematic behaviours, problematic people, or problematic social arrangements, the comparative risk assessment group can pretend that the problems just 'happened' and that no identifiable individuals or businesses caused them.

Ranking environmental problems rather than ranking problematic behaviours lets people avoid the reality that the problems were caused in part by social arrangements, such as the legal framework for corporations that favours decisions that bring short-term profits over decisions that protect public-trust resources such as air and water.

As a result, the solutions to the environmental problems ranked high by comparative risk assessment will be primarily technological and 'end-of-pipe' (correcting problems after they are created).

 Feedback

1   The argument is similar to ones you read elsewhere in this book, namely, that the act of doing risk assessments, comparative or otherwise, could be seen as a move which will necessarily lead to the legitimization of some hazards. It begs the question of whether the hazard, whatever its size, could be avoided in its entirety, and thereby undermines more thoughtful approaches that might be used.

2   There is no shortage of examples of where a narrowly selective approach to assessing individual risks could result in people taking their eye off the wider possibilities. What Mary O'Brien is proposing is a broader-based initiative that would permit a search for common roots of multiple problems, which might thus have a common solution. The problems associated with pesticide use in agriculture, for example, give rise to occupational hazards, chemical residues in foodstuffs, public health hazards, and ecological risks. All of these could be addressed by consideration of alternative agricultural practices which avoided or minimized pesticide usage, such as organic farming or integrated pest management.

3   It might well be that in some circumstances there is a preference by some stakeholders

for a narrower view to be taken. Some environmental health policies which would emerge from an O'Brien-style approach would require much more than, say, 'straight-forward' technological fixes. They might even require significant social change, and some would say, disruption. This could run into difficulties with all kinds of interests – professional, commercial, institutional and political. This is not to say that environmental health policy makers should avoid contemplating such options, though they should be aware that changes of that kind might introduce new health risks. As the British Medical Association (1998) has said, policies themselves may introduce their own health risks.

Alternatives assessment

In place of risk assessment, Mary O'Brien advocates what she calls alternatives assessment. Her argument is that while many of those who employ risk assessment for health policy purposes are doing their utmost to bring more evidence, candour, and realism to the decision process, the 'frame' may not be large enough. As she puts it:

Are you being allowed the room to learn about and calculate the pros and cons of all reasonable alternatives to the activity whose risk you are calculating? Risk assessment is, to some degree, dependent on the motives, assumptions, data bases, and intent of the risk assessors, but not as much as many people would hope. This is because risk assessment is fundamentally played out on a highly structured turf. The game played on this turf is to estimate, with more or less information and candour, how much of a hazardous activity is safe, insignificantly harmful, or acceptable. Alternatives assessment is a different game, played on different turf. The goal is to gather information from many people about the pros and cons of a variety of different paths to a goal. The goal itself is conceived as broadly as possible. If you are a skilled, honest, committed risk assessor (or policy adviser), you will be able to do much more to evoke needed information for good decisions about public health and the environment over on the turf of alternatives assessment.

The example of bovine growth hormone versus rotational grazing

Consider the case of recombinant bovine growth hormone (rbGH). This is a genetically-engineered growth hormone which can be injected into cows to increase their milk production. However, questions have been asked about its use. There is some evidence that it increases mastitis in cattle, which in turn increases dependence on veterinary drugs. This increases production costs, and traces of rbGH and the drugs may be passed on via milk to consumers. The benefits and disadvantages of rbGH compared to rotational grazing are given in Table 16.1.

Table 16.1 Some benefits and disadvantages of the use of rbGH versus rotational grazing

Issue	rbGH strategy	Rotational grazing strategy
Animal health	increased incidence of mastitis	better health than in a confined feeding system
Human health	more antibiotics needed to treat mastitis	no new health risks
Economics	competitive under conditions of high milk prices, low feed costs, low interest rates	competitive under conditions of low milk prices, high feed costs, high interest rates
Viability of rural communities	benefits larger units	promotes community self-reliance
Environment	higher use of nitrates and herbicides	less demand for fuel and chemicals

Source: Based on O'Brien (2000)

 Activity 16.2

Read the following edited passage from O'Brien which summarizes the pros and cons of rbGH and a radically different means of achieving similar results, rotational grazing, and also consider Table 16.1. In so doing:

1 Make a note of which issues might be dealt with in a conventional risk assessment and which might not.
2 Think of other issues which might be important to farmers and communities.
3 Identify any lessons about stakeholder consultation.

 Pros and cons of rbGH

We can also ask questions about alternatives to the risks of giving cows mastitis and feeding humans excess growth hormones. We could, for instance, compare reliance on rgBH with an alternative technology for increasing dairy farm profits: rotational grazing.

When grazing cows move from one pasture to another during a season, in essence they harvest most or all of their own food from perennial pasture crops. For most or all of the year, they are not confined in a barn or stockyard, to be fed crop plants that have been grown elsewhere and transported to them. In addition, by moving from pasture to pasture, the cows spread all or most of their own manure on the pastures during much of the year. In a confined feeding system, the manure becomes concentrated in one spot and must be spread mechanically by the farmer. If there is not enough land on which to spread manure, disposing of it is difficult. Nitrate-rich manure can pollute rivers and underground water supplies.

Rotational grazing and rgBH, then, are both technological approaches to milk production. Though not technically mutually exclusive, in practice, they are used separately.

Feedback

1 Some of the questions raised, like those about the incidence of mastitis and the transfer of traces of veterinary drugs to human consumers are the types of questions upon which a typical risk assessment would focus. However, issues of the effect upon farmers' lifestyles, the long-term impact upon pasture quality and ground water, and traditional community would likely be omitted. Changes in pesticide usage might also be overlooked, since they are an indirect consequence of rbGH usage.

2 Farmers and their dependants would probably also be concerned about the disruption of practices which may have shown themselves to be sustainable over long periods of time, and the potential threat this would pose to traditional lifestyles. Farmers would also become more dependent upon and therefore vulnerable to external suppliers, and this would introduce a quite different form of risk in a process sometimes known as 'risk substitution' (considered in Chapter 20).

3 The example draws attention to the fact that interventions of this kind – the potential substitution of traditional practices by modern technology – can have very diverse effects upon the ecosystem and upon community lifestyles and hence health and well-being. The implication is that consultation needs to be wide, in order to draw in as many stakeholders and affected parties as possible, so that these issues may be recognized and understood, and all available knowledge brought to bear.

Alternatives assessment and cost–benefit analysis

The debate over the relative merits of alternatives assessment and risk assessment also impinges upon cost–benefit analysis. Nicholas Ashford and Charles Caldart (1991), whose field is technology and public policy, have described three main advantages which are frequently assigned to cost–benefit analysis as a decision-aiding tool:

... first, cost–benefit analysis clarifies choices among alternatives by evaluating consequences in a systematic manner. Second, it professes to foster an open and fair policy-making process by making explicit the estimates of costs and benefits and the assumptions on which those estimates are based. Third, by expressing all of the gains and losses in monetary terms, ... cost–benefit analysis permits the total impact of a policy to be summarized using a common metric and represented by a single dollar amount.

Activity 16.3

In the following abridged extract, Mary O'Brien (2000) describes how alternatives assessment differs from this view of cost benefit analysis. As you read it, consider the following questions:

1 What are the strengths of the argument?
2 How might the argument be challenged?
3 Overall, where in your opinion does this leave risk assessment and cost benefit analysis?

Alternatives assessment

Alternatives assessment, like cost–benefit analysis, clarifies choices among alternatives by evaluating consequences in a systematic manner. The consequences (the costs and benefits) of alternatives assessment, however, can include issues of democracy, aesthetics, spiritual values, ethnic values, uncertainty, sense of community, and personal feeling as well as monetary consequences. What constitutes a 'systematic evaluation' of these consequences, of course, is a judgment. What may be crucially important to some may be marginal to others. Considering and comparing monetary consequences with aesthetic or cultural consequences may not appear as 'systematic' as comparing dollars to dollars, but it is more realistic than assuming that all significant consequences can be systematically translated into dollars. To speak of making decisions 'rationally' on the basis of money is to deny the reality that much that matters has no price tag.

Furthermore, like cost–benefit analysis, alternatives assessment fosters an open and fair policy-making process by making explicit the estimates of costs and benefits of the options being considered and the underlying assumptions. The costs and benefits considered in alternatives assessment, however, are more comprehensive. In alternatives assessment, costs and benefits are both monetary and non-monetary. An alternatives assessment to which the public contributes will be much more candid than a cost–benefit analysis, because many kinds of relevant pros and cons will be displayed for public consideration.

The third 'advantage' of cost–benefit analysis, i.e. the representation of the total policy or action by a 'common metric' of dollars, is not shared with alternatives assessment, because social and environmental realities cannot be reduced to a common metric such as dollars. Again, the tidy appearance of a common metric can be created only by denying social, political, spiritual, and environmental realities.

How, then, can we decide among the alternatives if we have to consider numerous groups and numerous factors, some of them financial, some cultural, some spiritual? The same way each of us makes decisions each day. Our decisions are sometimes based on sheer survival instinct, sometimes on overriding economic reasons, and sometimes on personal principles. Occasionally we choose one alternative because another simply doesn't seem the right one. Sometimes we choose an alternative extremely systematically, on the basis of explicit factors, after careful consideration of numerous options and after consultation with others.

Although both 'objective' cost–benefit analysis and messier alternatives assessment are political, cost–benefit analysis covers up the political nature of analysis with monetary numbers. Alternatives assessment forces the decision maker to assume responsibility for choosing among various explicit political and value tradeoffs. At the heart of good public decision making, governmental, business and corporate decision makers must take responsibility for their decisions that affect the public and the public's environment. They must be prevented from hiding behind 'dollar' numbers, just as they must be prevented from hiding behind 'risk' numbers.

 Feedback

1 The thrust of the argument is that, for some environmental policy decisions at least, there are wider, non-monetizable issues like spiritual and ethnic values that are important to people and which therefore need recognition and evaluation, and would benefit from public consultation. It is undeniable that things such as these are beyond monetization.

2 The message could be challenged as being self-evident. Welfare economists, for example, are at pains not to deny the existence of important, non-monetizable quantities and stress the need for these to be considered (e.g. Arrow et al. (1996), as discussed in Chapter 11). This, they stoutly argue, does not diminish the benefit to policy makers of the process of quantifying those inputs which are quantifiable. Not to do so would be to ignore potentially important information.

3 O'Brien's message, about the need to broaden the scope of risk assessment to think about alternatives, may be very useful in certain circumstances. In one sense it mirrors a key objective of SEA which was to turn attention to activities at the higher level of policy. This will not always be appropriate and could perhaps even lead to a paralysis of inaction, but it is arguably the case that decision making processes have had a tendency to be more restricted in scope than they should have been, so the message ought to be heeded. However, it might be felt that there is a danger that to go too far down that road could lead towards relativism, whereby anyone's opinion was as good as anyone else's, and the basis of decision making become more rather than less obscure. Most people, including the public, still support the use of quantitative inputs into decisions where it is relevant. This includes cultural theorists, and Mary O'Brien herself who says, in her book, that there is no need to oppose the assessment of risks, but rather that risk assessment should be extended to cover the risks and the benefits of a range of options.

Precaution and the precautionary principle

There is another argument with which students of environmental health policy must be familiar, and that is that if the 'Precautionary Principle' were followed, then there would be little need to rely upon risk assessment or other techniques of science for managing risk. We would merely avoid risks altogether, at least those which are anthropogenic, by not invoking them in the first place.

At the 1972 conference known as the London Dumping Convention, the environmental organization Greenpeace asserted the following:

This traditional 'permissive' approach does not represent a sound scientific approach to the protection of the environment. The existing body of scientific literature makes it clear that even the most sophisticated environmental impact assessment models contain substantial inherent uncertainty due to the overwhelming diversity and complexity of biological species, ecosystems, and chemical compounds entering the environment. What were once considered perfectly safe levels of particular inputs into the environment subsequently have been determined unsafe. The legacy of environmental degradation attests to this fact.

The precautionary argument sounds very sensible on the face of it, the Greenpeace argument has appeal, and there are undoubtedly cases where it would amount to good advice. However, from a policy perspective, the Precautionary Principle is less simple than it appears. To this effect, Per Sandin (1999) of Stockholm University has compiled a list of definitions as given by seventeen different agencies, a selection of which is shown in Table 16.2.

Table 16.2 Statements of the Precautionary Principle

Originating agency	How the Precautionary Principle is stated
UN, World Charter for Nature (1982)	Activities that are likely to pose a significant threat to nature shall be preceded by an exhaustive examination; their proponents shall demonstrate that expected benefits outweigh potential damage to nature, and where potential adverse effects are not fully understood, the activities shall not proceed.
Second International Conference on the Protection of the North Sea (1987)	Accepting that, in order to protect the North Sea from possible damaging effects of the most dangerous substances, a precautionary approach is necessary which may require action to control inputs of such substances even before a causal link has been established by absolutely clear scientific evidence.
Rio Declaration (1992)	In order to protect the environment, the precautionary approach shall be widely applied by States according to their capabilities. Where there are threats of serious or irreversible damage, lack of full scientific certainty shall not be used as a reason for postponing cost-effective measures to prevent environmental degradation.
Wingspread Conference (1998)	When an activity raises threats to the environment or human health, precautionary measures should be taken, even if some cause-and-effect relationships are not fully established scientifically. In this context, the proponent of an activity, rather than the public, should bear the burden of proof.
Bergen Ministerial Declaration (1990)	In order to achieve sustainable development, policies must be based on the Precautionary Principle. Environmental measures must anticipate, prevent and attack the causes of environmental degradation. Where there are threats of serious or irreversible damage, lack of full scientific certainty should not be used as a reason for postponing measures to prevent environmental degradation.
UK Government 1990 White Paper on 'Sustainable Development: the UK Strategy'	Where there are significant risks of damage to the environment the Government will be prepared to take precautionary action to limit the use of potentially dangerous materials or the spread of potentially dangerous pollutants, even where scientific knowledge is not conclusive, if the likely balance of costs and benefits justifies it.

Source: Based on Sandin (1999)

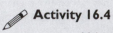 **Activity 16.4**

Make notes on the following:

1 The overall primary intention of the Precautionary Principle as revealed by the statements.
2 Any clauses that moderate the primary intention.

Feedback

1 The common intention is to tackle significant environmental threats, in advance, without waiting for complete scientific proof of cause and effect. The onus is placed upon polluters to provide evidence that their actions will not cause harm.

2 The UN World Charter for Nature contains the qualifying clause 'expected benefits outweigh potential damage', the Rio Declaration refers to the precautionary approach being applied by States 'according to their capabilities', and the UK Government moderates the principle with 'if the likely balance of costs and benefits justifies it'. All of these imply, with varying levels of intensity, that the Principle will still be subject to rational, economic analysis, involving cost–benefit considerations. It is also interesting to note that there is reference to 'absolutely clear scientific evidence' (North Sea Conference) and cause-and-effect relationships that are 'not fully established scientifically' (Wingspread Conference). This opens up an additional debate as to the meaning of the Principle. What qualifies as absolute evidence? Indeed, does science set out to produce absolute evidence? Even Newton's laws of motion and gravitation are not seen as absolute statements of unshakeable truth, but as hypotheses, and ones which have had to be modified as a result of work by Einstein.

Per Sandin (1999) goes on to analyse the Principle, as stated by the 17 agencies, in detail. He does this on the basis of the following general formulation of the Principle: '*If* there is (1) a threat, which is (2) uncertain, *then* (3) some kind of action (4) is mandatory.' Sandin observes that the phrases in the 17 statements which express these four dimensions vary in (a) precision and (b) strength, and that the weakest phrase is the one which determines the strength of the entire principle. Thus, in the formulation of the UK government the clause 'if the likely balance of costs and benefits justifies it' seriously weakens the 'action' dimension and hence the Principle itself. The Rio Declaration says nothing about what actions are to be carried out, but only that uncertainty is not a justification for inaction, amounting, as Sandin says, to a rule for legitimate discourse rather than for policy advice.

 Activity 16.5

The following abridged passage from Cass Sunstein (2002) describes the obvious emotional appeal of the precautionary principle, but also sounds a warning for policy makers. What is the basis of that warning and what is being implied as the remedy?

 Better safe than sorry?

All over the world, there is increasing interest in a simple idea for the regulation of risk: in the case of doubt, follow the Precautionary Principle. Avoid steps that will create a risk of harm. Until safety is established, be cautious. In a catchphrase: better safe than sorry. In ordinary life, pleas of this kind seem quite sensible. Shouldn't the same approach be followed by regulators (policy makers) as well?

There is some important truth in the precautionary principle. Sometimes it is much better to be safe than sorry. Certainly we should acknowledge that a small probability (say, 1 in 100,000) of a serious harm (say, 100,000 deaths) deserves extremely serious attention. It is worthwhile to spend a lot of money to avoid that risk. The fact that a danger is unlikely to materialise is hardly a good objection to regulatory controls. But everything depends on the size of the investment and the speculativeness of the harm. Unless the harm would be truly catastrophic, a huge investment makes no sense for a harm that has a one in one billion chance of occurring. Taken literally, the precautionary principle would lead to indefensibly huge expenditures, exhausting our budget well before the menu of options could be thoroughly consulted. If we take costly steps to address all risks, however improbable they are, we will quickly impoverish ourselves.

But there is a larger problem. The precautionary principle can provide powerful guidance only if we blinker ourselves and look at a subset of the harms involved. In real-world controversies, a failure to regulate will run afoul of the precautionary principle because potential risks are involved. But regulation itself will cause potential risks, and hence run afoul of the precautionary principle too. Hence the precautionary principle is literally paralyzing. It bans every imaginable step, including inaction itself.

 Feedback

Cass Sunstein's warning to policy makers is that even though precaution is a worthy consideration, it is still necessary to think carefully about resource allocation in the interests of public health and also to be aware that even precautionary interventions will, if thoroughly examined, be seen to generate secondary risks, just as medicines have side-effects, which introduces a logical inconsistency. The implication is that while being 'precautionary' has obvious political appeal and may at times be very sensible, analysis of costs and benefits is still required. In a nutshell, one might adapt Samuel Florman's (1987) aphorism, 'the precautionary principle is a sometimes useful tool that needs to be applied thoughtfully, not a machete to be flailed against every conceivable harm'.

Summary

Alternatives assessment seeks to extend the scope of risk assessment, which is still seen as necessary although of reduced importance, to cover the risks and benefits of a range of options to control target risks, some of which might involve social rather than technical change. It also seeks to encompass broader issues than those normally considered quantifiable in cost–benefit analyses. There are competing arguments about the novelty and utility of this – supporters of traditional cost benefit maintain that they do not at all preclude consideration of broader issues, nor seek to confine the agenda of environmental health policy makers.

Yet another challenge to conventional thinking comes from advocates of the 'precautionary principle'. Thoughtful analysis of this principle shows that it is interpreted in many different ways, some interpretations falling back on cost–benefit analysis, and some being much more demanding of evidence of no harm. It is evident that useful though the concept undoubtedly is in some circumstances, it needs to be handled carefully by policy makers.

References

Arrow K et al. (1996) *Benefit-Cost Analysis in Environmental, Health, and Safety Regulation*. Annapolis: The Annapolis Center.

Ashford N and Caldart C (1991) *Technology, Law and the Working Environment*. New York: Van Nostrand Reinhold.

British Medical Association (1998) *Health and Environmental Impact Assessment*. London: Earthscan.

Florman SC (1987) *The Civilized Engineer*. New York: St Martin's Press.

Graham JD and Wiener JB (1995) *Risk Versus Risk: Tradeoffs in Protecting Health and the Environment*. Cambridge, MA: Harvard University Press.

London Dumping Convention (1972) *Convention on the Prevention of Marine Pollution by Dumping of Wastes and Other Matter*. http://www.londonconvention.org/

O'Brien M (2000) *Making Better Environmental Decisions: An Alternative to Risk Assessment*. Cambridge, MA: MIT Press.

Sandin P (1999) Dimensions of the precautionary principle. *Human and Ecological Risk Assessment* 5(5): 889–907.

Sunstein CR (2002) *Risk and Reason: Safety, Law and the Environment*. Cambridge: Cambridge University Press.

SECTION 6

Making policy

17 From risk communication to participatory decision making

Overview

As the story unfolds, you will have noticed that more and more emphasis is being given to factors and concerns which some consider to have fallen outside the purview of traditional health policy decision making. One way of redressing this balance would be to find out what people care about in affected communities, what their problems are, and what insights they might have. In this chapter you will learn about how these ideas have impacted upon the traditional approach to decision making, and in particular the now perceived central role and importance of risk communication.

Learning objectives

By the end of this chapter, you will be better able to:

- **recognize and describe the role of risk communication in environmental health policy**
- **distinguish situations where different styles of risk communication are likely to be appropriate**
- **recognize the importance and nature of 'trust' as a determinant of communication style**
- **view the debate over risk communication and deliberation from atop the 'insight axis'.**

Key terms

Analytic-deliberation A process of decision making that involves both technical analysis and engagement with affected and interested parties.

Deliberation A reciprocal exchange of ideas between the public, interest groups and policy makers.

Governance The process of governing, or of controlling, managing, or regulating the affairs of some entity.

Risk communication Any meaningful communication between parties over matters of risk; not restricted simply to one-way communication.

Risk governance Encompasses the totality of participants, rules, conventions, processes and mechanisms concerned with the collection, analysis and communication of relevant information, and the making of policy decisions.

Changing styles of policy formulation and risk management

As you have progressed through this book you will have noticed an undercurrent of change in the way risks are perceived and managed and this is also increasingly reflected in the ways in which policies are formed. In fact, in many quarters, there is a strong trend towards involving stakeholders and other interested persons in decision making and policy formulation. This is reflected in the growing use of the term 'governance' over the last decade in many countries and international organizations. Governance refers to structures and processes that support *collective* decision making involving stakeholders and other interested parties. This trend has been brought about by a number of factors. Partly it is because there has been a growing feeling that many risks have not been well managed, and this has resulted in a loss of trust in conventional, political and technocratic approaches to decision making.

Additionally, a very public battle has been fought over how risk management, and policy decisions, should be made. As you read in Chapter 12, psychological studies have shown us that the wider public perceive risks in different ways from professionals, and in Chapter 13, on cultural theory, you encountered the notion of the legitimacy of the different world-views that are held by different groups. These disparate interpretations of the evidence, culminating in different ideas about what should be done, further reflected themselves in the proposed alternative strategies for addressing health risks, such as social impact assessment, strategic environmental assessment, health impact assessment, alternatives assessment, precautionary approaches, and so on. These alternatives seek, in part, to change the agenda, making it more encompassing of these other perspectives.

In 1995, Baruch Fischhoff, of Carnegie Mellon University, produced a very insightful account of how risk management, in its attitude to the wider community, had changed over the preceding 20 years. This trend is summarized in Table 17.1.

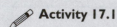 **Activity 17.1**

Examine Table 17.1 and make a note of what you consider to be its key features.

Table 17.1 The changing nature of risk management

All we have to do is get the numbers right.

All we have to do is tell them the numbers.

All we have to do is explain what we mean by the numbers.

All we have to do is show them that they've accepted similar risks in the past.

All we have to do is show them that it's a good deal for them.

All we have to do is be nice to them.

All we have to do is make them partners.

All we have to do is all of the above.

Source: Fischhoff (1995)

Feedback

Table 17.1 suggests that within the constituency being considered by Baruch Fischhoff, decisions about risk management had initially been made on the basis of technical considerations without a perceived need to engage with the wider community, a manifestly technocratic approach which could be described as paternalistic. As time passed, however, it became increasingly necessary to inform, explain, convince and win over those affected by the decision, culminating in a need to involve them, on an equal footing, as partners in the policy process. The last line of Table 17.1 is important too – it shows that the intention is that whatever the level of public involvement deemed appropriate, the technical input is undiluted and essential.

William Leiss (1996) has described the evolution of risk communication as having occurred in three phases. The first phase emphasized the necessity of conveying numerical information on risk to the general public and educating them over the need to accept the risk management practices of the respective institutions. If doubts remained, the main strategy was to argue that if people were willing to accept a voluntary risk of a certain magnitude, then they should accept an equal, or smaller, imposed risk. Of course, we now know from the psychometric paradigm that this is unlikely to work, and so a second stage of risk communication emerged in which the emphasis switched to persuasion and public relations exercises. This, essentially one-way communication process, was also found to be unconvincing for many people, and led to phase three which is often described as two-way communication in which experts are expected to learn from the public as well as the public from experts.

The analytic-deliberative process

This shift in opinion has had a very real impact upon the way in which the policy process is perceived in many countries and organizations. You will remember, from Figure 3.2, the classical approach to risk assessment and policy formulation as advised by the US National Research Council (NRC) in 1983, and which was fairly universally accepted at the time. This approach is best known for the way in which it drew a sharp distinction between risk assessment, seen as a technical function, and risk management, seen as a policy function which transcends science. However, as noted above, times and perspectives have changed, and the NRC has revised its proposed methodology accordingly, and this is illustrated in Figure 17.1.

Activity 17.2

Examine the process set out in Figure 17.1 and compare it with that in Figure 3.2. What is your opinion on the following?:

1   In what ways has it changed?
2   From what you have read in this book so far, what might be the justifications for the changes?

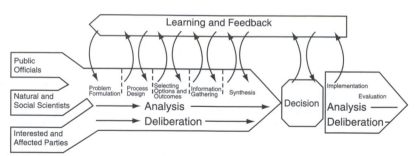

Figure 17.1 A schematic representation of the risk decision process
Source: NRC (1996)

 Feedback

1 There are several striking differences. Figure 17.1 clearly identifies the process of decision making as involving two interconnected threads, of which scientific analysis is one, and deliberation is the other (this is why the process is termed analytic-deliberation). Second, inputs to the process are shown as coming, not just from labora-tory and field measurements and other technical data, as indicated in Figure 3.2, but also from public officials and interested and affected parties. Furthermore, all parties are involved throughout the entire decision process in the exchange of ideas, information and opinions. Thus, everyone can (and should, according to this view) learn from every-one else at every stage of the process from framing to decision making.

2 Arguments in favour of this shift are of several types. In fact, Table 14.1 set out one way of looking at it. In Table 14.1 three justifications (normative, epistemological, and instrumental) were given for broadening participation, in that case in the EIA process, but the same can be applied to risk and policy decisions more generally. To recap, the justifications are that it is in the interests of democracy and because decisions are not value-free; that decision makers can learn from affected communities and stakeholders; and that broadening participation helps win acceptability of resulting policy decisions (Löfstedt 2005).

The NRC also redefines risk characterization. Their new definition is as follows:

Risk characterization is a synthesis and summary of information about a potentially haz-ardous situation that addresses the needs and interests of decision makers and of inter-ested and affected parties. Risk characterization is a prelude to decision making and depends on an iterative, analytic-deliberative process.

This definition too would appear to heed the concerns expressed by sociology, psychology, and exponents of the wider vision about how to go about engaging in policy decision making on health and the environment. It brings the affected communities into the decision process from the very beginning (the issue framing stage) and permits values to enter into the process.

This vision is reaffirmed in a recent White Paper on risk governance by the Inter-national Risk Governance Council (IRGC 2005) in Geneva (Figure 17.2).

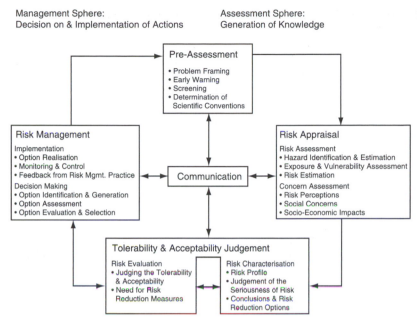

Figure 17.2 The IRGC risk governance framework

Source: IRGC (2005)

Activity 17.3

Study Figure 17.2 and consider the following:

1 The positioning and nature of risk communication.
2 How the standard model of risk assessment relates to the scheme.
3 The content of the pre-assessment phase.
4 How wider concerns are fed into and assessed by the process.

Feedback

1 Risk communication is two-way and permeates the entire cyclical process, from pre-assessment to decision making.

2 The standard model, as described in Chapter 3, is located in the risk appraisal phase.

3 The pre-assessment phase assumes greater importance and takes a broader view of issues and concerns of all those involved and potentially affected by the decision.

4 Concern assessment is an integral feature of the process, appearing as a part of the risk appraisal stage, and thus takes its place in this model alongside scientific, economic, social and cultural aspects. Concern assessment here refers to insights from risk perception studies and interdisciplinary analyses of the target risk's indirect social and economic implications.

Different decisions require different levels of engagement

All of this is not to say that every policy decision requires copious public engagement. This could be expensive, time-consuming, unwarranted and even counterproductive. Risk communication, especially dialogue-based risk communication, is not necessarily the be-all and end-all of risk management (Löfstedt 2005). It is necessary to proceed on a case-by-case basis, and the optimum approach will be influenced by the level of trust which exists between the affected community and the policy maker.

 Activity 17.4

Nonetheless, the following passage, adapted from the NRC (1996), explains in more detail the intention behind the new vision of decision making. As you read it, note how NRC distinguishes between different types of decision for the purpose of deciding upon the appropriate level of public and stakeholder engagement. Do you think that this would meet the objections of proponents of social impact analysis and alternatives assessment?

 A new vision of decision making

Different kinds of decisions require different kinds and levels of analysis and deliberation in support of risk characterization. For a series of similar risk situations, one might establish routines for risk analysis, characterization, and decision making that embody clear and consistent expectations about how the problem is defined, which options are to be considered, what kinds of evidence are to be considered, who is to participate in the process, and so forth. For novel, complex, or highly controversial risk situations – which often involve questions about major potential impacts and the equity of the distribution of risks and benefits – routines are likely not to be satisfactory. It is likely to be necessary to develop unique procedures for characterizing risk in these situations.

Some examples of procedures involving repetitive decisions are those for re-approving existing permissions for discharge of pollutants from industry, for testing new drugs prior to approval decisions, for issuing pre-manufacturing approval for the industrial production of new chemicals, and for deciding whether to exclude an individual from receiving a vaccine or giving blood. We do not mean to imply that all of the current procedures for these and similar decisions are appropriate; only that it is often appropriate to develop standard procedures. In fact, situations and knowledge change even for routine decisions, and standard procedures for risk analysis and characterization should be re-evaluated from time to time.

Risk situations need to be accurately diagnosed to determine whether existing standard procedures should be applied, whether new procedures need to be devised, whether additional information is needed to decide which approach to follow, and what extent and type of analytic and deliberative effort may be needed to reach such decisions. In medicine, experienced clinicians use a combination of knowledge, experience, and judgment to make diagnoses. The situation is closely comparable for those who must diagnose a risk situation and prescribe the appropriate kinds and level of analysis and deliberation needed and the appropriate breadth of participation.

Feedback

The NRC's recommendation is essentially that for routine, simple and uncontroversial hazards, the 'old' form of technocratic decision making, based upon routine procedures founded in experience and expertise may suffice, though periodic review of practices should still be undertaken. In the case of controversial or complex hazard situations, more emphasis should be placed upon engagement, consultation and deliberation.

It remains to be seen whether this recipe will satisfy everyone, including critics of the former risk assessment and EIA processes. However, it certainly looks like a step towards meeting those concerns which have been expressed. It should also be expected that not everyone will welcome this shift. For example, some people are firmly wedded, and believe very strongly, that the so-called rational approach to decision making is still the best way to make public policy decisions and that procedures which could dilute it will ultimately waste resources and cost lives (e.g. Breyer 1993). This is a dilemma with which environmental health policy makers will continually be confronted and to which there is not an easy answer. We will return to this.

Much thought has been put into the further refinement of this issue of when and how much engagement is desirable in policy decisions of various kinds. There are no hard and fast rules, every hazard and its context being unique in some way, but sociologist Ortwin Renn has produced a typology which is worthy of consideration. This is shown in Table 17.2, and in Figure 17.3 where it is referred to as the 'risk escalator'. Renn categorizes risk problems into one of four kinds: 'simple', 'complex', 'uncertain' and 'ambiguous' defined as follows:

1 *Simple*. Risk problems are ones for which the potential negative consequences are obvious, uncertainties are low, and the values involved are non-controversial. They are more-or-less straightforward to deal with and traditional methods of statistical analysis, use of goals determined by legislation, and conventional risk management techniques are applicable.

2 *Complexity*. Refers to the difficulty of identifying and quantifying causal links and specific observed effects. This may be due to interactions between agents (synergisms), delayed manifestation of effects, inter-individual variability of response, etc.

3 *Uncertainty*. Uncertainty is different from complexity but often results from an incomplete or inadequate modelling of cause–effect relationships. There are various sources: different vulnerabilities of targets; systematic or random errors in modelling; randomness of events; factors which are outside of the boundary of the modelled system but which might still be important; lack or absence of knowledge.

4 *Ambiguity*. This differs from the first two categories (which are epistemic in nature and can be reduced by improving existing knowledge and improving modelling tools). Ambiguity refers here to the different interpretations which may be placed upon accepted risk assessment results, a phenomenon described by cultural theory. There are two kinds of ambiguity. Interpretive ambiguity refers to different interpretations of a given result, whereas normative ambiguity refers to the matter of what is, or is not, tolerable.

Table 17.2 Risk characteristics and their implications for decision making

Knowledge characterisation	Management strategy	Appropriate instruments	Stakeholder participation
1 'Simple' risk problems	Routine-based: (tolerability/accept-ability judgement)	→Applying 'traditional' decision-making • Risk-benefit analysis • Risk-risk trade-offs	Instrumental discourse
	(risk reduction)	• Trial and error • Technical standards • Economic incentives • Education, labelling, information • Voluntary agreements	

2 Complexity-induced risk problems	Risk-informed: (risk agent and causal chain)	→Characterising the available evidence
		• Expert consensus seeking tools:
		  • Delphi or consensus conferencing
		  • Meta analysis
		  • Scenario construction, etc.
		• Results fed into routine operation
			Epistemological discourse

	Robustness-focussed: (risk absorbing system)	→Improving buffer capacity of risk target through: • Additional safety factors • Redundancy and diversity in designing safety devices • Improving coping capacity • Establishing high reliability organisations	
3 Uncertainty-induced risk problems	Precaution-based: (risk agent)	→Using hazard characteristics such as persistence, ubiquity etc. as proxies for risk estimates Tools include: • Containment • ALARA (as low as reasonably achievable) and ALARP (as low as reasonably practicable) • BACT (best available control technology), etc.	Reflective discourse
	Resilience-focussed: (risk absorbing system)	→Improving capability to cope with surprises • Diversity of means to accomplish desired benefits	

- Avoiding high vulnerability
- Allowing for flexible responses
- Preparedness for adaptation

| 4 | Ambiguity-induced risk problems | *Discourse-based:* | →Application of conflict resolution methods for reaching consensus or tolerance for risk evaluation results and management option selection
• Integration of stakeholder involvement in reaching closure
• Emphasis on communication and social discourse | Participative discourse |

Source: IRGC (2005)

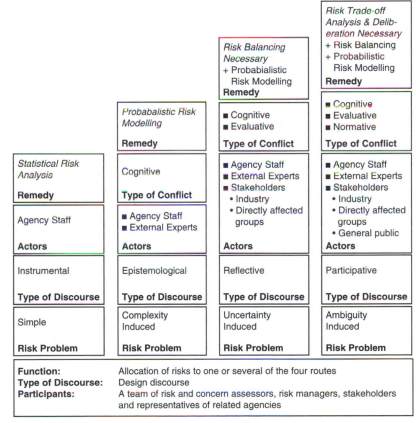

Figure 17.3 The risk management escalator and stakeholder involvement

Source: IRGC (2005)

Activity 17.5

Write down some examples of hazards which fall into each of the four categories.

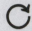 **Feedback**

Examples of hazards with complex characteristics would include large-scale industrial facilities and the synergistic effects of potentially toxic substances. Those with the characteristic of uncertainty would include volcanic eruptions, earthquakes, and the long-term effects of introducing genetically modified organisms into the environment. Examples of interpretive ambiguity include the possible effects of low doses of ionizing radiation and the use of antibiotics in animal husbandry. Normative ambiguities are associated with passive smoking, nuclear power, and genetically modified food.

To return to Table 17.2 and Figure 17.3, what is being proposed here is that for 'simple' risks which are relatively free of the above attributes, the management strategy may be routine and draw upon traditional decision making techniques of the types listed, with risk communication having an instrumental aim, that is, educational or to induce the desired response in affected parties. For 'complex' and 'uncertain' risks a different approach is needed, which may be directed either at the hazard itself, or those who are vulnerable. The following excerpt from IRGC (2005) explains:

For 'complex' and 'uncertain' risk problems it is helpful to distinguish the strategies required to deal with a risk agent from those directed at the risk-absorbing system (those affected or the environment): complex risks are thus usefully addressed on the basis of 'risk-informed' and 'robustness-focussed' strategies, while uncertain risks are better managed using 'precaution-based' and 'resilience-focussed' strategies. Whereas the former strategies aim at accessing and acting on the best available scientific expertise and at reducing a system's vulnerability to known hazards and threats by improving its buffer capacity, the latter strategies pursue the goal of applying a precautionary approach in order to ensure the reversibility of critical decisions and of increasing a system's coping capacity to the point where it can withstand surprises. Finally, for 'ambiguous' risk problems the appropriate strategy consists of a 'discourse-based' strategy which seeks to create tolerance and mutual understanding of conflicting views and values with a view to eventually reconciling them.

Figure 17.2 shows the centrality of risk communication in decision making.

 Activity 17.6

Write down what you believe to be the purpose(s) of communicating about risk.

 Feedback

Risk communication could have a number of purposes: enabling the public and stakeholders to understand the thinking behind decisions when they are not formally part of

> the process; helping people who are faced with risks by giving them factual information so that their choices are informed; fostering understanding of and hence tolerance for conflicting points of view; creating trust; enabling society to cope with and react to hazards of all kinds, whether acute or chronic in nature.

Approaches to risk communication

Risk communication is not a science but nonetheless, much has been learnt about its proper (and improper, i.e. how not to do it) conduct over the years, sometimes from bitter experience. Regina Lundgren (1994) has provided a valuable guide which should be consulted. This identifies three primary forms of risk communication which she calls care communication, consensus communication and crisis communication (Figure 17.4), each of which requires its own approach.

Care communication is about things like safety and environmental health. It can be subdivided into health risks such as AIDS, smoking, and exposure to environmental toxins, and, on the other hand, industrial exposure to chemicals or the risk of accidents. Consensus communication is about informing and encouraging groups to work together to decide on how to deal with a more complex hazard situation such as the Nepalese Bara Forest plan described in Chapter 14. Crisis communication refers to risk communication in the aftermath of major events such as the 2005 earthquake in northern Pakistan, the Indian Ocean tsunami of 2004, or major industrial accidents such as those at Bhopal, Chernobyl and Prince William Sound (the *Exxon Valdez*).

Of these, care and consensus communication are more likely to be of relevance to environmental health policy makers, and crisis communication will not be examined further here. Lundgren has described many of the factors which would-be care communicators should consider in preparing their communications:

- Principles of process
  - Know your communication limits and purpose.
  - Whenever possible, pretest your message.
  - Communicate early, often and fully.
  - Remember that perception is reality.
- Principles of presentation
  - Know your audience.
  - Don't limit yourself to one form or style of communication.
  - Simplify language and presentation but not content.
  - Be objective and not subjective.
  - Communicate honestly, clearly and compassionately.
  - Listen to specific concerns and deal with them.
  - Convey the same information to all interested parties.
  - Deal with uncertainty.
- Principles for comparing risks
  - Don't trivialize.
  - Use ranges where there is uncertainty.
  - Compare to Standards.
  - Compare to other persons' estimates of the same risk.

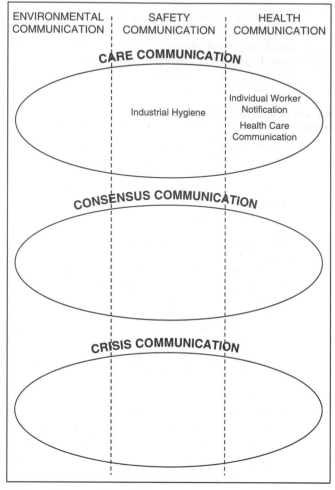

Figure 17.4 Three different realms of risk communication requiring different styles
Source: Lundgren (1994)

 Activity 17.7

1 What kind of communication is this primarily referring to?
2 In what circumstances might it be effective, and in what circumstances might it be unproductive?

Feedback

1 The recommendations primarily apply to what might be called 'top-down communication'. Scope is clearly permitted for interaction with audiences, but the emphasis is more on presenting and listening than on deliberating.

2 Top-down communication might well suffice and be the optimal approach in situations where there is trust between affected communities and policy makers, and where the hazards are familiar and non-controversial. Where trust has been lost, or hazards are complex or in some way ambiguous, the approach could lead to a further deterioration in relations.

The importance of trust

As Ragnar Löfstedt (2005) says, it is essential for policy makers to be aware of matters of trust when considering a communication strategy.

 Activity 17.8

In reading the following edited passage from his book, note the justifications given for encouraging stakeholder and public involvement, and reflect on their compatibility with the recommendations of Ortwin Renn as set out in the risk management escalator (Figure 17.3).

 Dialogue risk communication

The development of dialogue risk communication techniques was welcomed among both industry and regulators who were keen to learn how to increase public trust via more active engagement, as well as gain information on the affected citizens' preferences by involving them directly in the policy-making process. *It is because of its perceived ability to increase public trust that dialogue risk communication is very much in vogue.* Public/interest group participation is identified as important in rebuilding the legitimacy of the decision-making process.

 Feedback

The justifications, which would also apply to policy makers, are to increase trust, gain information on the interests of those affected, and secure legitimacy. These ideas are compatible with the right-hand column of Renn's risk management escalator (Figure 17.3), which deals with hazards involving questions of ambiguity and personal values.

Wouter Poortinga and Nick Pidgeon (2003) have analysed the nature of trust in some detail and proposed that it is more clearly understood if divided into a fourfold typology as shown in Figure 17.5, based on two dimensions, one being the general level of trust in policy makers and the other the level of belief, or scepticism, which surrounds a policy issue. They argue that it is important to distinguish between these different types of trust in any given situation. A potentially important matter for environmental health policy makers is that 'critical trust', for example, should not be confused with 'distrust', and may in fact be the *healthiest state of affairs* to exist between policy makers and their constituencies!

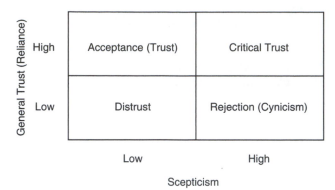

Figure 17.5 Four different kinds of trusts or mistrust

Source: Poortinga and Pidgeon (2003)

Deliberative approaches

Many kinds of deliberative decision making techniques have been developed. These range from focus groups, at the simple end, to much more elaborate methods including (citizens') juries, inquiries, (citizens') panels, joint-fact finding and much more. For more complicated and important issues, multi-stage techniques which involve technical experts and interested parties in carefully planned decision processes have been advocated. The Cooperative Discourse Model is one such approach which has been developed in particular by Ortwin Renn (Jaeger et al. 2001).

Deliberative approaches are, however, relatively new and largely experimental. They are not without their critics. The following passage is abridged from Löfstedt (2005) who summarizes the main concerns which have been aired:

📖 **Deliberative approaches**

. . . the deliberative process is a relative failure. There are several reasons for this. Research has shown that more deliberation in the policy-making process leads to public mistrust of policy-makers and the government as a whole; they only become more aware of how staid and ineffective bureaucrats can be. Some scientists and experts criticize deliberation, as they see no reason why the public, whom they view as under- or misinformed, lost, bewildered, overtly self-interested or simply apathetic, should participate in policy-making at all. In addition, the popularity of the deliberative process in the 1990s has resulted in more work for officials and a less efficient practice. Bureaucrats concerned about transparency have now begun to retreat from public meetings, favouring memos and informal discussions. The participatory process is also criticized for requiring the public to assimilate a lot of information about the particular issue being deliberated, which can lead to divergent rather than convergent views.

Henry Rothstein (2004) has examined a number of participatory decision processes in the United Kingdom, concluding that the broadening of participation *per se* does not necessarily produce more democratic or robust policy outcomes than closed processes, although it may have some limited value in improving public confidence in the regulatory regime.

The policy makers' dilemma

As you will have surmised, there is no simple recipe in this chapter for environmental health policy makers. Although techniques of risk communication are in vogue in some countries, the matter of when, where and how to apply them finds no simple answer. At the extremes, and to use a boxing analogy, in the red corner we have people who espouse 'technocratic risk management' and in the blue corner we have those who see any such approach as arrogant and inherently undemocratic. Once released into the ring, pitched battles are apt to break out.

US Supreme Court Justice Stephen Breyer (1993) is often cited as a defender of the 'red corner'. In his 1993 book, *Breaking the Vicious Circle*, he expressed concern about patchy and inconsistent approaches to risk assessment, and arguments involving the public who, he felt, were unable to judge risks reliably. The Breyer recipe was for a specific kind of group to take the lead in health policy decisions. This group would be 'mission oriented, seeking to bring a degree of uniformity and rationality to decision making in highly technical areas, with broad authority, somewhat independent, and with significant prestige'. To find an occupant of the opposite corner, one need look no further than Mary O'Brien (of Chapter 16) who describes Breyer's vision as 'nightmarish and undemocratic'.

With whom should the environmental health policy maker align herself or himself? Without wishing to raise your hopes unduly, perhaps the next chapter will provide some ideas, if not answers.

Summary

Risk communication is now firmly on the agenda of health policy decision makers, and the recognized need for it has influenced the decision making style of many countries and agencies. It is not, however, a panacea, and it is necessary to think carefully about the appropriate style of communication, whether top-down, participatory, or something in-between. An important factor in deciding what is necessary in a given circumstance will be the nature and complexity of the hazard being considered, and the issue of trust. Trust is itself not a straightforward concept and needs to be examined carefully on a case-by-case basis. Although the current fashion in some sectors is very much communication-oriented, not everyone is convinced and important questions remain unanswered.

References

Breyer S (1993) *Breaking the Vicious Circle: Towards Effective Risk Regulation*. Cambridge, MD: Harvard University Press.
Fischhoff B (1995) Risk perception and communication unplugged: twenty years of process. *Risk Analysis* 15(2): 137–45.

IRGC (2005) *Risk Governance: Towards an Integrated Approach*. Geneva: IRGC. Available at: www.irgc.org

Jaeger CC, Renn O, Rosa EA and Webler T (2001) *Risk, Uncertainty and Rational Action*. London: Earthscan.

Leiss W (1996) Three phases in risk communication practice, in Kunreuther H and Slovic P (eds) *Annals of the American Academy of Political and Social Science: Challenges in Risk Assessment and Management*. Thousand Oaks, CA: Sage.

Löfstedt R (2005) *Risk Management in Post-Trust Societies*. New York: Palgrave Macmillan.

Lundgren R (1994) *Risk Communication: A Handbook for Communicating Environmental, Safety, and Health Risks*. Columbus, OH: Battelle Press.

National Research Council (1996) *Understanding Risk: Informing Decisions in a Democratic Society*. Washington, DC: National Academies Press.

Poortinga W and Pidgeon NF (2003) Exploring the dimensionality of trust. *Risk Analysis* 23(5): 961–72.

Rothstein H (2004) Precautionary bans or sacrificial lambs? Participative risk regulation and the reform of the UK food safety regime. *Public Administration* 82(4): 857–81.

18 | Philosophy, politics and prejudice

Overview

By now you will be aware, if you were not before, that all is neither simple nor calm within the world of environmental health policy. There are sharp divides between those who advocate so-called 'rational' models of policy formulation and those aligned to models with a wider 'social' emphasis. There is also disagreement over who should make policy decisions, and especially the extent to which the public should be invited to participate. While the near-term existence of a formula for resolving these disputes is doubtful, and hence you might think there are grounds for pessimism, an alternative strategy is to try to understand the roots of these disagreements. Already you are familiar with two sociological theories, cultural theory and the psychometric paradigm, which offer valuable insights. In this chapter you will further examine the rifts from a philosophical and political perspective. The aim is to achieve maximum insight into these fundamental differences so you are better equipped to recognize available choices. You will also think about the matter of 'prejudice' and its contribution to decision making and, in conclusion, the essential and unforgiving challenge of environmental health policy formulation.

Learning objectives

By the end of this chapter, you will be better able to:

- **recognize the underlying philosophical and political roots of policy options**
- **understand the political nature of differences in opinion over the various approaches to environmental health policy**
- **discuss the nature of prejudice and its role in decision making**
- **be aware of the unavoidable challenges faced by environmental health policy advisers.**

Key terms

Communitarianism A philosophy that values communities and resists the idea that individuals and free market exchanges are the key social institutions.

Egalitarianism A moral perspective emphasizing equality of people.

Utilitarianism (welfarism) Based on the notion that society's interests are best served through the maximization of individual utilities.

Approaches to the formulation of health policy

Wider reflection upon how society functions with respect to decision making and policy formulation has pointed to four basic needs: these are for efficiency, effectiveness, social cohesion, and legitimacy (Renn 2005). Efficiency is achieved via economic balancing; effectiveness is about ensuring that measures adopted will, with reasonable expectation, yield the desired result, and derives from expert knowledge and science (the technocracy); social cohesion refers to the need to incorporate human values and fairness, and, as you saw in the previous chapter, can be addressed by consultation and deliberation. It concerns the communication and exchange of interests such that disparate values are recognized and fairness is achieved. Legitimacy is about compatibility with legal requirements and political culture and emanates from the political system. Within modern societies, these four systems are maintained by economics, science, social systems and politics (Figure 18.1).

Most environmental health policy decisions take input from all four of these systems. This is partly at least because health policies designed to help one community are likely to have impacts, possibly adverse, on others (BMA 1998; Graham and Wiener 1995). In real societies all things are coupled together in some way, people and institutions alike, and cannot be considered as independent atomistic entities as in the idealized RAP model. It is also because each system is regarded as having its own strengths and weaknesses, as summarized for three of the systems, in Table 18.1, so by using them all there is more chance of success. As you read through Table 18.1 you should recognize all the entries. This is because you have already studied these three systems: in Chapters 3 to 7 you encountered the technocratic approach to policy formulation as taken by science; in Chapters 8

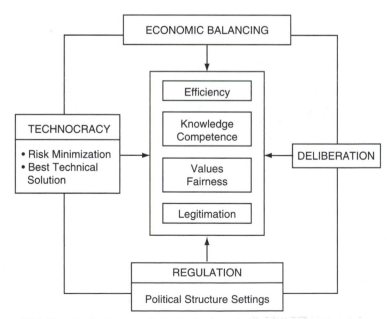

Figure 18.1 Four idealized approaches to policy formulation

Source: © Ortwin Renn. Reproduced with permission.

Table 18.1 A comparison of the benefits and disadvantages which have been attributed to three different policy approaches

Policy approach	Cited benefits	Cited disadvantages
Technocratic	– increases benefits of environmental health policies – gives credibility to policies – reduces dependence on moral and legalistic arguments – the scientific approach has produced huge health benefits – there is public support for the use of science in policy decisions	– sometimes seen as arrogant and undemocratic – unlikely to work if trust is low – not all issues are about purely science (e.g. Bara Forest) – knowledge is far from perfect and uncertainty may be significant – can be seen as a way of permitting the continuance of risks rather than avoiding them – experts are fallible and results can be manipulated – even scientific decisions involve value judgements – risk assessment tends to introduce conservative bias (by repeatedly erring on the safe side)
Economic	– the economic (market-based) approach is more efficient than command and control – resources are saved – compliance costs are reduced – provides an incentive to develop better control mechanisms – exposes the conservative biases to which risk assessments are prone – exposes the biases to which the public and policy makers are vulnerable (e.g. that there is more concern for highly visible and dramatic risks than those which cause most harm etc)	– the process is elitist and answers 'how safe is safe enough?' without direct recourse to the affected public – equity issues are not considered, nor are many other factors which people care about, mainly because they cannot be quantified – it assumes that economists are right in the way they measure public preferences (WTP etc) – cost–benefit analysis downplays unquantifiable risks – ignores social values e.g. altruism – tends not to handle uncertainty well – the monetary valuation of health is challenged – measuring and aggregating public preferences is difficult, even for economists
Consultative/ deliberative	– strengthens democracy by informing and involving the public – gives legitimacy to decisions – brings on board issues of equity and other non-quantifiable but important factors – does not subjugate the issue of what level of risk is tolerable to a mathematical formula – makes use of publicly-held knowledge as well expert knowledge – dialogue is better than top-down risk communication or no communication at all – increases trust	– open to exploitation – may subvert democracy – can diminish trust – may lead to relativism – costly and time consuming – experimental and unproven – requires the public to assimilate large amounts of technical information

Source: Based partly on Löfstedt (2005)

to 10, the economic approach; and in Chapters 11 to 16, social factors increasingly played a role including, in Chapter 17, the extra step to participatory and deliberative decision making.

What has not so far been discussed is the political-philosophical dimension. In discussing this fourth system, the emphasis is going to be upon exploring how different political philosophies underlie different approaches to decision making. You will recall from Chapter 13 how cultural theory offered an insightful explanation of why different groups respond differently to similar information. Another window on this phenomenon can be elicited by examining the political roots of policy making. First though, you need to think about the role of values in decision making. The philosopher David Seedhouse, whose primary interest is health care, has this to say:

Health promotion is thought, by many theorists and practitioners, to be based primarily, or even entirely, on evidence and facts. But this is a crucial mistake. Health promotion is much more to do with values (and politics) than even the most radical health promoters realise.
(Seedhouse 2000)

Since health care policy and environmental health policy have much in common, what would be true for one would presumably be true for the other. But is it true?

What motivates environmental health policy?

Seedhouse proposes that while most policy makers believe that when it comes to policy it is the evidence which comes first, the truth is in fact the reverse. There is thus a false perception that environmental health policies are formed in this order:

1　There is evidence of preventable environmental health problems (this evidence is either factual or highly probable – and it is the main driver of policy).
2　There are strategies designed to deal with the preventable problems (there is usually a *choice* of strategy, and values may be *one* of the factors influencing the choice).

And in recent years:

3　There are additional strategies meant to protect the environment itself even where there is no evidence of human health problems.

But instead, environmental health policies are formed in this order:

1　Policy makers hold particular values and political philosophies.
2　There is evidence of preventable environmental health problems (this evidence is selected according to values and political philosophy – even the decision to call something an environmental problem or not is thus inspired though this is not to say the evidence is entirely shaped by prejudice – there can be better and worse reasons to intervene.
3　Strategies designed to deal with preventable environmental problems are selected according to values, political philosophy and evidence – the key questions are: do we think this ought to be done and will it work?

And in recent years:

4　There are additional strategies to safeguard the environment even where there are no existing human health problems.

Activity 18.1

In policy decisions, is it the case that 'facts always speak for themselves'? Or is it true that policy makers interpret evidence according to their particular values and political philosophies?

 Feedback

It is evidently the case that environmental health promotion is not factual but essentially value-based. This is demonstrated by the fact that priorities differ between different administrations, between different groups, in different geographical locations, and at different times, even when essentially the same problems are faced.

The political underpinnings of environmental health policies

Once it is conceded that environmental health policy is inspired by political values, it becomes essential to ask 'what values?' It is fortunate that, just as cultural theorists decided that four world-views were sufficient for the purposes of their theory (and even one of those, the fatalist view, was not much used), the reality is that there are not that many core sets of political values to choose from.

In fact, within this book, you have encountered in very general terms just three political bases. Table 18.2 summarizes, in a much simplified form, what these are about, under the three headings of 'rational health policy', 'environmental health policy', and 'social health policy'. Rational health policy would be anchored in techniques like risk assessment and potential Pareto optimization, and is generally assumed to be objective and evidence-based because it aims to improve measurable aspects of people's lives. On the other hand, social health policy sees life (society) as more complex and seeks to improve people's lives by social change. It is particularly concerned with social inequalities, whereas rational health policy is more interested in getting an appropriate health return for its investment. The third type is environmental health policy. This comes in many shades, from relatively mild to 'deep Green', and is directed more towards the protection of the ecosystem as a whole than to people, though it may also be a part of the intention that people will benefit if the ecosystem is healthy. Of course, the true picture is much more complicated than this, nevertheless, it can be used as a starting point for understanding some of the controversies which permeate environmental health policy formulation.

Table 18.2 indicates how each of these three policy types can be traced to an underlying political philosophy. For example, you can trace how rational health policy emanates from a political philosophy of prudence, utilitarianism, and preservation of the status quo. Essentially, it is conservative in nature. Similarly, links can be made between social health promotion and different varieties of social democracy and egalitarianism. This political outlook is inspired by the essential equality of all people, and the importance of communities as well as individuals.

Table 18.2 A simplified analysis of the possible political roots of three different approaches to environmental health policy

'Rational' health policy	'Environmental' health policy	'Social' health policy
Environmental health exists in the absence of measurable disease, illness, injury and handicap	Environmental health is about the well-being of the ecosystem	Environmental health exists in the absence of threats to health
Environmental health problems are bad of themselves	If the ecosystem is healthy people will also have the greatest chance to be healthy too	Environmental health threats are bad in themselves
Environmental health problems are also disruptive and incur losses of working time and medical costs	Threats to the ecosystem are also bad because they pose risks to other creatures	Environmental health threats are also bad because they pose risks to peoples' potentials
Environmental health risks can be managed by appropriate science-based interventions		Environmental health threats are unequally distributed across social groups
		The causes of environmental health threats are manifold but sometimes they are the result of how people have to live
Environmental health interventions should be instigated where health benefits exceed costs	The avoidance of threats to the environment is our responsibility. We should 'tread lightly on the earth.'	Where environmental health problems are the result of broader social issues health policy should consider social change
PRUDENCE UTILITARIANISM PRESERVATION OF THE STATUS QUO CONSERVATISM	ENVIRONMENTALISM	EGALITARIANISM SOCIAL DEMOCRACY SOCIALISM

Source: Adapted from Seedhouse (2000)

✎ Activity 18.2

As you read the following edited passage by John Graham (2001) on the economic evaluation of health interventions and the political roots of decision making (specifically, liberalism, which includes egalitarianism and utilitarianism) think carefully about the following questions:

1 In Chapter 9 you encountered a framework for decision making in the context of the control of radiation exposure, summarized in Figure 9.8, and in Chapter 10 you read about the 'tolerability of risk' framework, summarized in Figure 10.2. Have these frameworks been influenced by political philosophies, and if so, which?

2 In Chapters 14 and 16, you read about several alternatives to the Rational Actor Paradigm for determining environmental health policy, including health impact assessment, social impact assessment, and alternatives assessment. Can the evident contest between these models and, say, RAP, be attributed to different underlying political philosophies and, if so, how?

Political roots of decision making

There are three major philosophical traditions that have influenced political thinking in the English-speaking world: liberalism, utilitarianism, and communitarianism.

'Liberalism' refers to both libertarians, who seek to protect and expand the private sphere of life by defining those 'negative' rights of citizens that government may not violate, and egalitarians, who pursue more fairness and equality in life by defining 'positive' rights of citizens that government is obliged to supply. For strict liberals of either stripe, there is little interest in economic efficiency since the formulations of rights determine what a society should do to advance the welfare of citizens. Strict commutarians, who believe that public policy should evolve out of community-defined values (whether ethically or religiously defined), have also expressed little interest in economic efficiency. Of course, 'strict' liberals and communitarians, defined as those who have no interest in other perspectives, are few in both number and influence and thus there is interest throughout the world in practical tools to operationalize utilitarian thinking, at least as a partial contribution to public policy.

The philosophical perspective of utilitarianism has been defined as involving some calculation of 'the greatest good for the greatest number'. Cost–benefit analysis, in particular, arose out of efforts to translate social utilitarianism into a practical tool for public policy makers. From this body of scholarship arose a definition of 'economic efficiency'. In the most ambitious thinking of early writers, the economic-efficiency test was proposed as a necessary and sufficient condition for public policy intervention. This ambitious position is no longer favored due to growing philosophical and political interests in fairness as well as efficiency. For example, an environmental health policy aimed at a low-income population that is both effective and inexpensive might still be judged 'economically inefficient' if the beneficiaries, due to their low ability to pay, do not express sufficient interest (as defined by WTP) in the benefits of the measure. These kinds of fairness concerns have led to the viewpoint that economic efficiency should be a contribution to public policy choice but efficiency should not be considered a necessary or sufficient condition for public intervention. One of the most perplexing challenges is to determine how much weight to give to efficiency and fairness in making public policy decisions.

Feedback

1 Both of these frameworks for decision making contain a strong element of utilitarianism. This comes in via the concepts of ALARA and ALARP which are about optimization and seeking the greatest good for the greatest number i.e. economic efficiency. However, the frameworks also incorporate dose and risk limits above which no person should be exposed, and in this way an element of liberalism-egalitarianism is

introduced. This is why, in the right-most column of Table 8.1, where these frameworks lie, they are referred to as 'hybrid' approaches.

2 It should be clear that whereas RAP is rooted in the left-hand column of Table 18.2 and is therefore underpinned by utilitarian beliefs and conservatism, social impact assessment is more readily associated with the right-hand column and hence egalitarianism and social democracy. Health impact assessment, at least as described in Chapter 14, remains essentially a RAP-style approach, merely aiming to incorporate health considerations more overtly into the environmental impact assessment process. Alternatives assessment, on the other hand, is much more concerned with social, political, spiritual and environmental priorities than with economic optimization, and seeks to take a wider societal view of environmental health policy and challenge the status quo. It is therefore more strongly associated with the right-hand column of Table 18.2, and, as expressed in Chapter 16, may have some anchorage in the central column too.

Environmental health programmes

Just as tools for policy makers may carry with them a political ideology, so do all environmental health programmes.

Table 18.3 lists 18 targets of the Kazakhstan Ministry of Health. Although information is limited, you might conclude from this list that these targets are of different kinds, being anchored in different political philosophies and hence requiring different approaches to implementation.

Table 18.3 Targets of the Kazakhstan Ministry of Health (1998)

1	To improve the environment and prevent morbidity relating to the environment
2	To provide drinking water
3	To eradicate poliomyelitis by the year 2000, to reduce diptheria, pertussis and measles; to reduce viral hepatitis morbidity and mortality
4	To reduce maternal mortality and prenatal morbidity
5	To improve the reproductive health of the population
6	To promote children's health and reduce the mortality rate for children under 5
7	To reduce morbidity, mortality and disability from tuberculosis
8	To increase knowledge about sanitary hygiene; to develop new population behaviour patterns and healthy lifestyles
9	To develop modern medical technologies and equipment
10	To further develop the primary health care sector
11	Form markets in health services (including privatization and non-state actors) and improve their quality
12	To shift from in-patient to out-patient principles of treatment
13	To achieve adequacy, efficiency and cost effectiveness
14	To lower the dependence of Kazakhstan on imported drugs (pharmaceuticals)
15	To reform training of specialists within the medical education system to meet international standards
16	To develop medical science
17	To reform organizational and administrative bodies within the health care system
18	To attain sustainable financing

Activity 18.3

Examine the list and make a note of the more indicative tendencies of this kind, i.e. whether some objectives are more clearly motivated by utilitarianism as opposed to egalitarianism or environmentalism and vice versa.

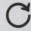 **Feedback**

The first targets on the list are primarily egalitarian in nature, whereas from No. 9 onwards the tendency is for a 'rational' approach to health policy. Thus, the early targets on the list talk about 'reducing', 'preventing' and 'improving' health without reference to efficiency and item 8 refers to the intention to 'develop new population behaviour patterns and healthy lifestyles', a clear indication of a preference for social health policies. Items 11, 13 and 16, in contrast, are clear indicators of an interest in a 'rational' style of health policy, and some of the other items may be too, depending upon how they are implemented.

The unavoidable role of prejudice

This chapter has emphasized that people's choices about which health policies to pursue and how, are based upon values as well as, and arguably more than, facts. Further, whereas you have read about the importance of psychology and culture in shaping opinions, here the emphasis has been on the role of political philosophies. This is not at all to say that scientific evidence is unimportant, for most people would agree that it is. To deny the contribution of science would be to descend into the fruitless morass of relativism. So, to make sense of the world, it is necessary to collect the evidence and interpret it, the latter requiring a belief system or philosophy against which to perform this task. However, it will often be the case that better or worse interpretations can be identified, and sometimes it will be possible to say that interpretations are completely right or completely wrong, in either an analytic or a moral sense. The implication for policy makers is that they should not be unaware of the roots of their choices and that, from time-to-time at least, they should re-examine them. As John Adams might say, if you aspire to making policy, you should endeavour to move up the insight axis (of Figure 13.4), and that means seeing through the political biases or prejudices of others as well as your own.

 Activity 18.4

The following adapted passage from David Seedhouse describes three principal types of prejudice. In reading, make a note of which is an appropriate form and which is not for an environmental health policy maker. Does this offer any explanation of the rifts between rational, social and environmental health policies?

Three types of prejudice

The situation is confused because of a failure to make the following distinctions. There are at least three different kinds of prejudice:

1. Necessary prejudice. This is any belief on which a person grounds her reasoning and/or actions. Prejudice, in this sense, is a prerequisite for any thoughtful action (for anything other than instinctive or intuitive behaviour). In this sense prejudice is 'prejudgement' without which it is not possible to think about anything. Thus my belief that the sun will rise tomorrow is a prejudice, it is a prejudice that my friends are trustworthy, and a prejudice of mine that fire burns wood. Unless I judge these things to be true I cannot act in some of the ways I do act. I might be wrong, but my (normally intuitive) pre-judgement is that I am right.

A *necessary prejudice* may be either inescapable (in the sense that in everyday life it is simply absurd not to assume that heavy objects fall to earth, for instance) or chosen (I choose to believe in the fidelity of my friends). Whatever the case, a prejudice should be considered necessary if it appears to be just not possible to act without recourse to it.

2. Blinkered prejudice. This is a belief which is held, by the believer, to be an objective truth such that the person who holds it will not alter or abandon it whatever the evidence or whatever the argument he hears against it. Such a prejudice can be held about matters of evidence – for instance, a person might believe absolutely that wood always burns when exposed to flame – or about matters of value – for instance, a person might believe absolutely that smoking cigarettes is always an unhealthy behaviour.

It is possible to make a further distinction in this category too: a *blinkered prejudice* can be held either knowingly or unknowingly. Most of us, I assume, hold countless prejudices which, although not *necessary* in the above senses, it has never occurred to us to examine (one extreme example is that certain races are inferior to others: you might be able to come up with personal examples of your own, perhaps with help from someone who knows you well). And we also hold many prejudices which we have deliberated over, but which we have decided need no further reflection (one example might be that the rational health policy model is inadequate).

3. Reasoned prejudice. This is a position arrived at through reflection on either evidence or values or both, is open to revision, and is a prejudice which the holder is continually prepared to question and to defend if he believes it to be defensible.

 Feedback

Sooner or later prejudice has to enter into any deliberation about environmental health policy, so environmental health policy will *always* be open to dispute. Thus, the contest between rational, social and environmental policy models is a fact of life and not just a temporarily unresolved difference of opinion. Cultural theory tells the same story. Ask yourself: how can anyone seek to promote environmental health without holding a prejudice of some kind? Can anyone promote health without having an opinion about whether one way of living, and one way of intervening, is better than another? It is not possible. The evidence does not speak for itself, but, remember, *neither* is it mute.

It should also be obvious that only the first and third of the above forms of prejudice should be countenanced by participants in environmental health policy.

Remaining dilemmas of environmental health policy makers

Aside from the prejudices of policy makers, what about those of the public? Environmental health policy makers are often in the position of making decisions which affect the well-being of possibly many people to a far greater extent than they affect themselves. These decisions can be ethically challenging because the stakes are high and the value issues complicated. In this book you have encountered a number of reasons why policy makers should incorporate public values and perceptions into their decisions. However, while it may well be that incorporating public input into policy decisions will usually lead to better decisions, this is not guaranteed.

An insightful paper by Sarah Lichtenstein and colleagues (1990) posited a number of questions which would continue to tax decision makers dealing with public health. These, and their answers, can be summarized briefly:

What should be done if the public object to the use of Decision Analytic techniques for policy formulation?

People may object to the formal structuring and codification of complex decisions, but this should be rejected firmly because social decisions are made under conditions of resource constraints and trade-offs, like it or not, must be acknowledged even if it is claimed that they are morally repugnant.

What risk attitude (risk averse, prone or neutral) should policy makers take?

Policy makers should be avowedly risk neutral because the more compelling moral obligation is to save as many lives as possible. If there are additional costs associated with catastrophic events, these should be incorporated as additional factors in an analysis and not as some form of risk aversion.

Which concerns should be included in an analysis?

All attributes that are important to the affected people should be included, unless they are illegal, outside the policy makers remit, or of the 'not in my back yard (NIMBY)' variety.

What if people are misinformed?

To inform them would be a solution but may not always be possible or, if trust is low, achievable. This is a difficult situation, the proper answer to which is uncertain.

What if the individual preferences of the public differ from the societal policy perspective?

Again, this is a difficult scenario and one which would have to be analysed on a case-by-case basis.

Do people really want what they say they want?

This presents further difficulties. Answers to questions may, for example, reflect the way a question is worded or framed, and are in any case hypothetical and not necessarily reflective of what people might really want, for example, if they had to pay for it ('expressed preferences' are cheap). Policy makers should be hesitant, even about apparently strongly-held public positions, until they are confident.

You would be correct in deducing from this that there are still very real challenges for environmental health policy makers. The following passage, adapted from their paper, acknowledges the difficulties and provides a supportive message:

Our purpose is to encourage others to join us in thinking about the ethical problems faced by policy makers in making their decisions when their views differ from those of the affected public. We feel compassion for the decision makers, struggling to do the right thing in difficult circumstances. We want our policy maker to be intellectually well armed with an understanding of decision analysis sufficient to ensure that complex social problems can be viewed from a broad, consistent perspective. We also want our policy maker to have a backbone, able to go against (while never ignoring) public desires, and a heart, caring for and respecting (but not always acquiescing to) public views. This is a tall order, we admit. These are tough problems, unavoidably so.

Summary

Environmental health policy decisions are driven as much if not more by values than by evidence. These values can be shown to be anchored in different political philosophies, and in turn offer an explanation of the on-going contests between rational, social and environmental models of health policy. The selection of any particular environmental health intervention will, in part, be based upon prejudice. Of the various forms of prejudice around, only some should be harboured by policy makers. These are necessary prejudice and reasoned prejudice, and even these should be reviewed periodically. Environmental health policy makers should expect to continue to be confronted with many technical and ethical dilemmas. It is the nature of the job and is unlikely ever to go away.

References

British Medical Association (1998) *Health and Environmental Impact Assessment*. London: Earthscan.

Graham JD (2001) Economic evaluation of injury control: alternative perspectives, in *Proceedings of the Third International Conference on Measuring the Burden of Injury*. Baltimore, MD: US Department of Transportation.

Lichtenstein S, Gregory R, Slovic P and Wagenaar WA (1990) When lives are in your hands: dilemmas of the societal decision maker, in Hogarth RM (ed.) *Insights in Decision Making*. Chicago: University of Chicago Press.

Löfstedt RE (1995) *Risk Management in Post-Trust Societies*. New York: Palgrave Macmillan.

Renn O (2005) The challenge of integrating deliberation and expertise: participation and discourse in risk management, in MacDaniels T and Small M (eds) *Risk Analysis and Society: An Interdisciplinary Characterisation of the Field*. Cambridge: Cambridge University Press.

Seedhouse DF (2000) *Health Promotion: Philosophy, Prejudice and Practice*. New York: Wiley.

SECTION 7

Initiatives – local to global

19 | Issues of local policy

Overview

The final section of this book is about past and current environmental health policy initiatives. While you will read about some of the many schemes which have been devised, the intent is not to give a detailed résumé, but to identify issues which are deserving of thought from an environmental health policy perspective. Many initiatives are driven by genuine concerns and this is what places them on the political agenda, but to carry them through to fruition requires more than a vision. It requires a will to make things work and staying power. There are also many questions which should be asked of policies. What is their exact purpose? What motivates them? What tangible evidence is there that they are working? Can their hoped for effectiveness be measured? How much evidence should you expect? In the first of these closing chapters, the focus is upon local initiatives.

Learning objectives

By the end of this chapter, you will be better able to:

- discriminate between fact and fancy in the presentation of programmes
- reflect upon the nature and quality of evidence
- recognize the merits of programmes that can legitimately claim to be evidence-based but not necessarily disown those which cannot
- decide where the appropriate balance lies between the desire for proof and the benefits of acting
- avoid over-selling your case.

Key terms

Agenda 21 A global plan led by the United Nations which seeks to integrate environmental, social and health issues into decision making.

Capacity 21 and 2015 Capacity-building programmes which support Agenda 21 and the quest for sustainability.

Social capital The institutions, relationships, and norms that shape the quality and quantity of a society's social interactions.

Policy routes

Very broadly speaking, there are two principal routes for instigating environmental health policies. One is via so-called top-down initiatives which emanate from central or regional governments or international organizations and which influence central planning. The other is through stimulating bottom-up or 'grassroots' activities. Grassroots activities may of course arise spontaneously, but there has been an acceptance that the gains which are potentially achievable by this route can be realized more quickly with appropriate help from the centre.

You will also have sensed, in reading through this book, the gradual shift from the way of thinking which saw problems as being solved by a centralized expert-driven technocracy to a process in which the wider community could usefully participate. Likewise, the view has taken hold that local communities, by making use of their own 'social capital' could do much to help themselves, and might even provide a solution to larger-scale problems if effective measures were replicated across other communities. The term 'social capital' is interesting. Unlike the economist's concept of 'human capital', social capital could be described as the sociologist's counterfoil, namely, it is about the importance of social networks and trustworthiness in a properly functioning society. You might recall the argument over RAP, which sees society as a collection of 'atomistic' individuals pursuing their own individual interests, a view rejected by sociology. Thus, a RAP society may contain many virtuous but isolated individuals, but could still be low in social capital. To paraphrase the World Bank, social capital refers to the institutions, relationships, and norms that shape the quality and quantity of a society's social interactions. Social capital is not just the sum of the institutions which underpin a society – *it is the glue that holds them together*. In this way social capital is said to be important because it allows citizens to resolve collective problems more easily, it oils the wheels that allow communities to advance smoothly, and it widens awareness of the interlinking of people's interests (Putnam 1995, 2000).

A further important cross-cutting theme for policy makers is that of sustainability which adds further impetus but also complications. The classic definition of sustainability originates from the 1987 Brundtland Report of the World Commission on Environment and Development, entitled *Our Common Future*: 'Sustainable development is development which meets the needs of the present generation without compromising the ability of future generations to meet their own needs.'

Sustainability implies the need to conserve both energy and material resources, to maintain biodiversity and to reduce pollution to stabilize planetary conditions. Note, however, that sustainability is notoriously difficult to quantify and there is no consensus on what constitutes a sustainable state for the world. Currently the richest 20 per cent of the world's population consume 80 per cent of its resources. This puts the burden of responsibility for change on the rich countries, though it is clear that rising living standards in the rest of the world will have a large impact on resource consumption. This raises both economic and ethical issues but unfortunately these two disciplines are uncomfortable companions.

Agenda 21 and Capacity 21

Agenda 21 was designed by the United Nations as a comprehensive plan of global action to be applied nationally and locally by organizations of the UN, governments, NGOs and other groups in every area in which people impact upon the environment, with the aim of integrating environmental and developmental issues, including health, into decision making. An explicit requirement is to involve communities, businesses, the health sector and other partners in finding solutions to health and environmental problems. On the website of the UN Division for Sustainable Development (UNDSD) can be found a full statement of the intent of Agenda 21. Chapter 6 of the statement deals with the protection and promotion of human health and begins as follows:

 Community involvement in Agenda 21

Health and development are intimately interconnected. Both insufficient development leading to poverty and inappropriate development resulting in over-consumption, coupled with an expanding world population, can result in severe environmental health problems in both developing and developed nations. Action items under Agenda 21 must address the primary health needs of the world's population, since they are integral to the achievement of the goals of sustainable development and primary environmental care. The linkage of health, environmental and socio-economic improvements requires inter-sectoral efforts. Such efforts, involving education, housing, public works and community groups, including businesses, schools and universities and religious, civic and cultural organizations, are aimed at enabling people in their communities to ensure sustainable development. Particularly relevant is the inclusion of prevention programmes rather than relying solely on remediation and treatment. Countries ought to develop plans for priority actions, drawing on the programme areas in this chapter, which are based on cooperative planning by the various levels of government, non-governmental organizations and local communities. An appropriate international organization, such as WHO, should coordinate these activities.

There are six associated programme areas: primary health care, communicable diseases, vulnerable groups, the urban health challenge, and risks from environmental pollution, and hazards. All of these are of interest to environmental health policy makers, though here, for illustrative purposes, the last is selected. The *basis for action* is expressed as follows:

 Basis for action

In many locations around the world the general environment (air, water and land), workplaces and even individual dwellings are so badly polluted that the health of hundreds of millions of people is adversely affected. This is, *inter alia*, due to past and present developments in consumption and production patterns and lifestyles, in energy production and use, in industry, in transportation etc., with little or no regard for environmental protection. There have been notable improvements in some countries, but deterioration of the environment continues. The ability of countries to tackle pollution and health problems is greatly restrained because of lack of resources. Pollution control and health protection measures have often not kept pace with economic development. Considerable development-related environmental health hazards exist in the newly industrializing countries. Furthermore, the recent analysis of WHO has clearly established the interdependence among the factors of health, environment and development and has revealed that most countries are lacking such integration as would lead to an effective pollution control mechanism. Without prejudice to such criteria as may be agreed upon by the international community, or to standards which will have to be determined nationally, it will be essential in all cases to consider the systems of values prevailing in each country and the extent of the applicability of standards that are valid for the most advanced countries but may be inappropriate and of unwarranted social cost for the developing countries.

 Activity 19.1

The above passages describe the basis for action on environmental pollution and hazards. What are seen as the causes of health and environmental problems, what are seen as the solutions, and by what philosophy or culture might these views be inspired?

 Feedback

Problems are attributed to insufficient and inappropriate development, over-consumption, and an expanding population. The solution is seen as lying in intersectoral efforts and cooperative planning which enable people to bring about sustainable development. The reference to population growth is reminiscent of the hierarchist view of global problems as described by cultural theorists in Chapter 13. According to that analysis, the 'population story' emerges from hierarchically structured institutions, and the heroes would be those organizations with the capacity (technical knowledge) and 'right' sense of moral responsibility to sort it out. Nonetheless, this apparent hierarchist tendency is softened by the evident desire to involve communities, though how this links to the end game of sustainable development is not explained.

 Activity 19.2

The following extract describes the objectives and activities of this part of the programme. What is the nature of the approach to environmental health improvement?

 Reducing health risks from environmental pollution and hazards (Agenda 21)

Objectives

The overall objective is to minimize hazards and maintain the environment to a degree that human health and safety is not impaired or endangered and yet encourage development to proceed. Specific programme objectives are:

(a) By the year 2000, to incorporate appropriate environmental and health safeguards as part of national development programmes in all countries;

(b) By the year 2000, to establish, as appropriate, adequate national infrastructure and programmes for providing environmental injury, hazard surveillance and the basis for abatement in all countries;

(c) By the year 2000, to establish, as appropriate, integrated programmes for tackling pollution at the source and at the disposal site, with a focus on abatement actions in all countries;

(d) To identify and compile, as appropriate, the necessary statistical information on health effects to support cost/benefit analysis, including environmental health impact assessment for pollution control, prevention and abatement measures.

Activities

Nationally determined action programmes, with international assistance, support and coordination, where necessary, in this area should include:

(a) Urban air pollution:
   i   Develop appropriate pollution control technology on the basis of risk assessment and epidemiological research for the introduction of environmentally sound production processes and suitable safe mass transport;
   ii Develop air pollution control capacities in large cities, emphasizing enforcement programmes and using monitoring networks, as appropriate;

(b) Indoor air pollution:
   i   Support research and develop programmes for applying prevention and control methods to reducing indoor air pollution, including the provision of economic incentives for the installation of appropriate technology;
   ii Develop and implement health education campaigns, particularly in developing countries, to reduce the health impact of domestic use of biomass and coal;

(c) Water pollution:
   i   Develop appropriate water pollution control technologies on the basis of health risk assessment;
   ii Develop water pollution control capacities in large cities;

(d) Pesticides:
   Develop mechanisms to control the distribution and use of pesticides in order to minimize the risks to human health by transportation, storage, application and residual effects of pesticides used in agriculture and preservation of wood;

(e) Solid waste:
   i   Develop appropriate solid waste disposal technologies on the basis of health risk assessment;
   ii Develop appropriate solid waste disposal capacities in large cities;

(f) Human settlements:
   Develop programmes for improving health conditions in human settlements, in particular within slums and non-tenured settlements, on the basis of health risk assessment;

(g) Noise:
   Develop criteria for maximum permitted safe noise exposure levels and promote noise assessment and control as part of environmental health programmes;

(h) Ionizing and non-ionizing radiation:
   Develop and implement appropriate national legislation, standards and enforcement procedures on the basis of existing international guidelines;

(i) Effects of ultraviolet radiation:
   i   Effects of ultraviolet radiation: Undertake, as a matter of urgency, research on the effects on human health of the increasing ultraviolet radiation reaching the earth's surface as a consequence of depletion of the stratospheric ozone layer;
   ii On the basis of the outcome of this research, consider taking appropriate remedial measures to mitigate the above-mentioned effects on human beings;

(j) Industry and energy production:

   i   Establish environmental health impact assessment procedures for the planning and development of new industries and energy facilities;

   ii Incorporate appropriate health risk analysis in all national programmes for pollution control and management, with particular emphasis on toxic compounds such as lead;

   iii Establish industrial hygiene programmes in all major industries for the surveillance of workers' exposure to health hazards;

   iv Promote the introduction of environmentally sound technologies within the industry and energy sectors;

(k) Monitoring and assessment:

Establish, as appropriate, adequate environmental monitoring capacities for the surveillance of environmental quality and the health status of populations;

(l) Injury monitoring and reduction:

   i   Support, as appropriate, the development of systems to monitor the incidence and cause of injury to allow well-targeted intervention/prevention strategies;

   ii Develop, in accordance with national plans, strategies in all sectors (industry, traffic and others) consistent with the WHO safe cities and safe communities programmes, to reduce the frequency and severity of injury;

   iii Emphasize preventive strategies to reduce occupationally derived diseases and diseases caused by environmental and occupational toxins to enhance worker safety;

(m) Research promotion and methodology development:

   i   Support the development of new methods for the quantitative assessment of health benefits and cost associated with different pollution control strategies;

   ii Develop and carry out interdisciplinary research on the combined health effects of exposure to multiple environmental hazards, including epidemiological investigations of long-term exposures to low levels of pollutants and the use of biological markers capable of estimating human exposures, adverse effects and susceptibility to environmental agents.

 Feedback

The approach is technocratic and inspired by RAP-like thinking.

There are copious references to hazard surveillance, monitoring networks, risk assessment, epidemiological studies, health risk analysis, well-targeted strategies, and the quantitative assessment of health benefits and costs associated with different strategies. Nonetheless, it would appear from the preamble that ideas from social health policy, and of social capital, have been knocking on the door. Indeed, under the heading of 'Capacity building', the following passage occurs:

Each country should develop the knowledge and practical skills to foresee and identify environmental health hazards, and the capacity to reduce the risks. Basic capacity requirements must include knowledge about environmental health problems and awareness on the part of leaders, citizens and specialists; operational mechanisms for intersectoral and intergovernmental cooperation in development planning and management and in combating pollution; arrangements for involving private and community interests in dealing with social issues; delegation of authority and distribution of resources to intermediate and local levels of government to provide front-line capabilities to meet environmental health needs.

This desire to promote local activities in support of sustainable development was furthered by the creation, by the 1992 UN Conference on Environment and Development (UNCED), of Capacity 21. Capacity 21, now superseded by Capacity 2015, sought to find the best ways of achieving sustainability and meet the goals of Agenda 21. During its time Capacity 21 worked with over 75 developing and transitional countries to promote capacity-building activities which would address environmental degradation, social inequity and economic decline. The kinds of activities encompassed by Capacity 21 are described on a country-by-country basis on the UNDP's website (UNDP 2006).

 Activity 19.3

If you can visit the UNDP's Capacity 21 website (UNDP 2006) and, taking the widely acclaimed Costa Rican programme as an example, make notes of how that programme strove to meet the three principles of Capacity 21, that is, to ensure participation of all stakeholders in programme development, implementation, monitoring and learning; to integrate economic, social and environmental priorities within national and local policies, plans and programmes; and to provide information about sustainable development to help people make better decisions.

 Feedback

These objectives were addressed by generating a new National Environmental Action Plan and setting up a National Council of Sustainable Development (CONADES) to foster collaboration between government and society. Major efforts were made to create public awareness of the work and encourage local participation, also seen as a means of safeguarding the programme into the future. A network of national organizations was also established for the purpose of ensuring that sustainability remained a priority. Technical expertise was garnered from a team of national experts providing input on green accounting systems, biodiversity and climate change etc.

It should be borne in mind that while the international community has given its support to Agenda 21 because of its strong commitment to the idea of local involvement, not all programmes have been seen as successful as that of Costa Rica, and some have been regarded as failures. While this could be put down to teething problems, there remain real questions about how Agenda 21 works and whether its benefits could ever be measured. Nor is it fully understood how or even if sustainable development can truly be achieved (notwithstanding this, there appears to be a consensus that it can only occur at global level if first it takes hold at the local level).

Other health-promoting initiatives

Consistent with Agenda 21, a plethora of programmes, some informal and many associated with the WHO, have been instigated. These come under such names as Healthy Cities, Healthy Islands, Healthy Villages, and Safe Communities.

Activity 19.4

Do you live in a city, a village, or on an island? Think about what your vision of a 'healthy city/village/island' would be and answer the following questions:

1 What are the most important things you would want done to make it better?
2 How could this be achieved?
3 Is your choice of what to do based more on evidence or more on values?
4 Would you anticipate any opposition, and if so from where?
5 Would you use scientific evidence to support your case?

Feedback

Because of the range and unpredictability of answers, only some very general pointers can be given. What you should notice though, in trying to do this exercise, is that your values are crucial determinants of what you want to do and how you propose to go about it. Otherwise, how could you say that your healthier vision was the best that could be achieved? Is your vision of a place which maximizes equality and in this way reduces health differentials, or is it one which tries to create greater wealth through work opportunities, thereby improving health and well-being? Or do you aspire for a simple(r) more environmentally-friendly way of life? Would you achieve your goal by a bottom-up, community-led approach involving social change, or would a top-down imposition of 'rational' health advancement measures be your preference? As you know, all these approaches indicate political leanings of one kind or another. There-fore, in normal circumstances, you should expect opposition from those who have other leanings and beliefs about how things work and should be done. As for the matter of evidence, many things that we think, or are firmly convinced, are worth doing are very hard to prove when it comes down to it. Some of the remaining case histories in this chapter are evidence of this. Much, it seems, rests on what is believed to be true.

Safe communities – an example

Following on from the launching by the WHO of the Healthy Cities initiative in 1988, the Safe Communities movement was also adopted the following year with the Karolinska Institutet in Sweden acting as Collaborating Centre. The Safe Community concept focuses upon injury prevention and relies upon community-based initiatives. By 2004, 83 communities from Scandinavia to China, South Africa and New Zealand had been designated as Safe Communities (Rahim 2004).

Activity 19.5

As shown in the ROAMEF cycle of Figure 8.1, an important task for policy makers, though one which is often neglected because it is difficult and time-consuming, is the *evaluation* of interventions. In the first of two passages (adapted), Carolyn Coggan and colleagues (2000) describe their evaluation of a community-based injury prevention programme in Waitakere, New Zealand known as the WCIPP. In reading the first passage, make notes on the following:

1 How did the authors go about evaluating the programme's effectiveness?
2 What did they conclude was good about the WCIPP?

 ### The WCIPP evaluation study

Evaluation of the community-based injury prevention project was conducted over a three year period (1995–1997). The overall goal was to ascertain the process and impact of the WCIPP model and the progress towards a reduction in injuries within Waitakere. The evaluation was also designed to provide information relevant to policy development.

Process evaluation activities conducted throughout the entire three-year pilot phase included analysis of project documentation to obtain information relating to implementation; participant observation at monthly management group meetings and official presentations organised by the WCIPP; regular telephone communication and six monthly key informant interviews with each of the three coordinators; and six monthly key informant interviews with either management group members and key council staff or representatives from community organisations in Waitakere.

For the *outcome evaluation* a quasi-experimental research design was used. A comparison population (147,000) was matched to the intervention population (155,000) on a number of relevant variables (demographic characteristics, new housing developments, road safety, and safer community (crime prevention in New Zealand) coordinator positions in both councils. Three primary sources of data were collected: injury statistics; a pre-post intervention telephone survey of Waitakere and the comparison population; and a pre-post survey of Waitakere and the comparison population organizations.

Morbidity data for admissions to public and private hospitals were obtained from the New Zealand Health Information Service National Minimum Dataset for the years 1989–98. Records for patients who had been hospitalised overnight as a result of receiving an injury were extracted for the areas of Waitakere, greater Auckland, and the comparison community. Injury hospitalisation rates were calculated from 1991 and 1996 census figures. Analysis of trends was conducted for all age groups. As childhood injuries were a particular focus for the WCIPP, a separate analysis was carried out for children aged 0–14.

To assess the *impact of the WCIPP on organisations*, a questionnaire was developed to cover awareness of the project and injury prevention and to assess changes in safety policies and practices. A total of 144 organisations were contacted in Waitakere and in the comparison community in 1995 and 1997. Organisations were matched and included the local council, preschool centres, schools, alcohol and drug prevention agencies, police, fire service, and rest homes.

Outcome evaluation

So far as injury rates were concerned, Waitakere was the only community to show a decrease in injury hospitalisation rates in both 1997 and 1998 (Figure 19.1). Rates for the comparison community increased in 1996/1997 but decreased slightly in 1998. Rates for

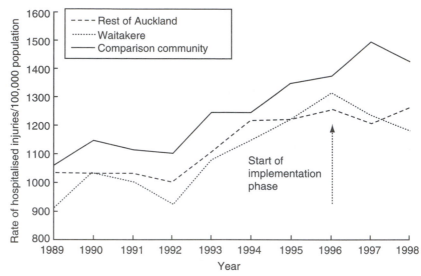

Figure 19.1 Injury hospitalisation rates for all ages

Source: Coggan et al. (2000)

the rest of Auckland increased in 1996, decreased slightly in 1997, and then increased again in 1998. There was no significant difference between the communities in the change in slopes during the intervention/post-intervention period. Compared with pre-intervention and comparison data, a highly significant increase in awareness of injury prevention was found. Increases in awareness of the WCIPP and injury prevention among Waitakere organisations were also evident.

In summary

In this first outcome evaluation of the WHO Safe Communities model in New Zealand, significant reductions in the rate of injury hospitalisations for children were achieved in Waitakere, whereas the comparison community showed an increase. This is an important finding as child safety was one of the major campaigns conducted by the WCIPP. Reductions in serious injuries have not yet been able to be demonstrated in similar projects conducted in Australia.

The WCIPP was not able to demonstrate significant reductions in injury hospitalisations rates for all age groups. However, it is very encouraging that Waitakere was the only community to show a decrease in injury hospitalisation rates for two subsequent years (1997/98).

The WCIPP was unable to replicate findings of significant reductions in self reported injuries for either adults or children. It is unclear why this has occurred. One explanation could be that the activities of the WCIPP have resulted in more Waitakere residents being aware of injury as a public health issue and this knowledge resulted in a more accurate recall of self reported injury. The WCIPP was successful in raising awareness of injury prevention among individuals and community organisations.

Feedback

1 The approach had three strands. One was to look at essentially administrative aspects of the project, the second was to look at injury trend data, and the third was to search for behavioural changes in organizations. Importantly, and as a means of trying to increase confidence that any observed trends in Waitakere were attributable to the intervention, the study also looked at similar communities and institutions outside of the WCIPP so that comparisons could be made.

2 The strongest conclusion statistically was that there was an increase in awareness of injury prevention. The actual description of the injury trend data in the communities is not very convincing since only for children was a favourable trend discovered and the time frame was short (Figure 19.1). The authors were nonetheless quite confident that the programme had had a positive effect upon child injury hospitalizations.

The second passage is from a review, by Per Nilsen (2004), in which he evaluates 16 community injury prevention programmes from around the world. Nilsen concludes as follows:

Ultimately, this study demonstrates the current difficulties of finding scientific evidence to support the community-based approach to injury prevention programming. Because of the inherent complexity of multistrategy and multitarget programs, and the interdependency between contextual, structural, and process aspects, it is still difficult to provide solid evidence describing the factors that are most important to achieve program effectiveness. Some of the problems of identifying key success factors are due to meagre descriptions of community characteristics and conditions, insufficient assessment of structural program components, and failure to establish process–outcome relationships. To advance the understanding of community-wide injury prevention programs, the evaluations that accompany them must develop in complexity.

These findings are clearly more sobering. Nilsen points to the difficulties, and sometimes even the dangers (since some of the interventions had apparently had adverse effects), of community intervention programmes. He found in particular that the most successful programmes had occurred in more homogeneous communities (in terms of ethnicity and socio-economic status). Programmes, it seemed, had to be adapted from community to community and country to country, and there was not a standard WHO Safe Community model which would work everywhere.

Healthy villages – an example

The Healthy Village programme is an extension of the WHO's Healthy Cities project that was initiated in Sarawak in 1994, sharing in common the view that attempts to improve health outcomes need to focus not just on health but also on social, environmental and economic factors. Andrew Kiyu carried out an evaluation of this programme in 2003. The following paragraph summarizes the scope of the Healthy Village programme in the Kapit District of Sarawak, the method of evaluation, and the outcome of their investigation. Immediately after this is another passage which records the limitations of the study.

Activity 19.6

In reading the paragraphs by Andrew Kiyu and colleagues, comment on the nature of the evidence presented and its limitations. What should be done?

 Healthy Village programme in Sarawak

Sarawak, Malaysia, has a large population of ethnic minorities who live in longhouses in remote rural areas where poverty, non-communicable diseases, accidents and injuries, environmental hazards and communicable diseases all contribute to a lower quality of life than is possible to achieve in these regions. To address these issues and improve the quality of life for longhouse people, the Kapit Divisional Health Office implemented the World Health Organization's Healthy Village programme in 2000. An evaluation was undertaken in 2003 to determine physical and behavioural changes resulting from the programme. The main changes evaluated were those involving smoking habits, exercise habits, health screening, fire safety, environmental improvements and food preparation and hygiene. A qualitative evaluation was conducted using participant observation and key-informant interviews, focus groups and observation. Results indicate that the programme is inspiring changes in various behavioural and physical characteristics of the study population. It is clear that the Healthy Village programme is a widely accepted way of improving health outcomes in longhouses, and that it is succeeding in making beneficial health changes.

The methods of analysis used in this study had a variety of limitations mainly because the analysis took place 2 years after the introduction of the programme and because of the absence of ongoing evaluation and a fixed evaluation framework. Baseline data on a variety of health issues was often either unavailable or incomplete making the ability to determine significant short-term changes in some but not all cases difficult, and in turn making it hard to determine significant long-term changes as well.

Despite these difficulties, there was strong and consistent evidence obtained from interviews of changed practices and improved health conditions since the implementation of the Healthy Village programme. This was reinforced by evidence of partial success from newer entrants to the programme that were at intermediate stages in implementation, and further reinforced from the baseline situation observed in non-participating villages.

 Feedback

The evidence is clearly observational and largely qualitative. No pre-intervention baseline had been established, and the work which was done was relatively *ad hoc*. Evidence from similar communities that were non-participating, and from those new to the programme, apparently supported the proposition that beneficial changes had occurred as a result of the programme. What else could be done? Realistically it may be that not much more could be done in the circumstances. Sarawak is probably not as well established in terms of health surveillance as some other localities and the cost and time to set up such systems might be better spent on other activities. And quantitative data are not always what they are said to be. Human observation and insight are in some circumstances, especially relatively novel situations, better at identifying and recording what is important.

Summary

The political view is now widely held that community-level participation in policy making, and the empowerment which this seemingly implies, have the potential to be a major factor in improving health and achieving sustainability. As a consequence, many countries have risen to the challenge posed by Agenda 21 and similar initiatives. While this belief may well one day be proved to have been correct, at present it appears to be more hypothesis than fact. Environmental health and social issues are intertwined in complex ways which are seldom fully understood. On the other hand, pressure always exists to show that programmes satisfy the three goals of effectiveness, efficiency and equity. In the absence of a deeper understanding of how complex social systems work and a lack, in most settings, of appropriate baseline data and surveillance systems, environmental health policy makers need to tread carefully between underselling their programmes and making claims which might not stand up in the cold light of day.

References

Coggan C, Patterson P, Brewin M, Hooper R and Robinson E (2000) Evaluation of the Waitakere community injury prevention project. *Injury Prevention* 6: 130–4.

Kiyu A, Steinkuehler AA, Hashim J, Hall J, Lee PFS, Taylor R (2006) Evaluation of the healthy village program in Kapit District, Sarawak, Malaysia. Health Promotion International 21(1): 13–18.

Nilsen P (2004) What makes community based injury prevention work? In search of evidence of effectiveness. *Injury Prevention* 10: 268–74.

Putnam RD (1995) Bowling alone: America's declining social capital, *Journal of Democracy* 6(1): 65–78.

Putnam RD (2000) *Bowling Alone: The Collapse and Revival of American Community*. New York: Simon and Schuster.

Rahim Y (2004) Safe community in different settings. *International Journal of Injury Control and Safety Promotion* 12(2): 105–12.

Seedhouse DF (1997) *Health Promotion: Philosophy, Prejudice and Practice*. New York: Wiley.

United Nations Development Program (2006) *Capacity 21 in Costa Rica*. Available at: http://www.capacity.undp.org/index.cfm?module=Projects&page=Project&ProjID=725

20 | Issues of global policy

Overview

Protecting the global environment is now a major challenge of public policy and international diplomacy. Notwithstanding the fact that there are serious matters which need attention, the purpose of this chapter is to highlight the complex issues involved in designing and promoting appropriate environmental health interventions. The examples taken are stratospheric ozone deletion and greenhouse gas emissions. You have already encountered the global climate change story, analysed from the perspective of cultural theory, in Chapter 13. The emphasis here is upon barriers to the creation of international agreements and treaties.

Learning objectives

By the end of this chapter, you will be better able to:

- **recognize the propensity of policy interventions to create new risks**
- **analyse environmental health policy interventions for the creation of new risks**
- **be aware of situations that could give rise to unduly narrow policy perspectives and so result in missed opportunities**
- **understand difficulties inherent in designing international environmental agreements.**

Key terms

Countervailing risk A newly created risk that results from action to reduce a target risk.

Risk trade-off The change in the portfolio of risks that occurs when a new risk is generated (knowingly or inadvertently) by an intervention to reduce a target risk.

Risk trade-off analysis An organized approach to identifying countervailing risks and assessing the balance of the full risk portfolio associated with a policy intervention.

Target risks The risk that is the primary focus of an environmental health intervention.

The threat to the stratospheric ozone layer

Although the naturally occuring gas ozone is present in small concentrations throughout the atmosphere, most ozone (about 90 per cent) exists in the stratosphere at a height of between 10 and 50 km above the surface of the Earth. For us, this ozone layer performs the essential task of filtering out most of the sun's biologically harmful ultraviolet radiation (UV-B). In 1985, scientists identified a thinning of the ozone layer over the Antarctic during the spring months which became known as the 'ozone hole'. Scientific evidence shows that human-made chemicals are escaping into the atmosphere and are responsible for the creation of the Antarctic ozone hole. Ozone depleting chemicals (ODC) have been used in many products which take advantage of their physical properties, e.g. chlorofluorocarbons (CFCs) have been used as aerosol propellants and refrigerants.

CFCs are harmful to ozone because they are broken down by sunlight in the stratosphere, producing halogen atoms (e.g. chlorine and bromine), which subsequently destroy the ozone through a complex chemical reaction. For reasons to do with the meteorology of the stratosphere, ozone destruction is greatest at the South Pole, though it does occur elsewhere. Stratospheric ozone levels have been observed to be decreasing annually since the 1970s. Mid-latitudes have experienced greater losses than equatorial regions. In 1997, the Antarctic ozone hole covered 24 million km^2 in October, with an average of 40 per cent ozone depletion and ozone levels in Scandinavia, Greenland and Siberia reached an unprecedented 45 per cent depletion in 1996 (Europa 2005).

Environmental and health effects of ozone depletion

The amount of UV reaching the Earth's surface has been shown to correlate with the extent of ozone depletion. In 1997, UV-B levels at the Earth's surface continued to rise at a rate of 2 per cent per annum. Increased UV levels at ground level pose risks to human health, including increases in the incidence of certain types of skin cancers, cataracts and immune deficiency disorders. Depletion of stratospheric ozone also alters the temperature distribution in the atmosphere, resulting in indeterminate environmental and climatic impacts.

Future perspective

Despite existing regulation of ODS, there continues to be severe ozone depletion and maximum stratospheric levels of chlorine and bromine are predicted to occur only during the next decade. Without further measures, the ozone hole will continue to exist beyond 2050. However, the success of the Montreal Protocol has already been observed in terms of changes in the concentrations of man-made chlorine-containing chemicals in the lower atmosphere, which means that the rates of release of ODC to the atmosphere have been reduced:

The Montreal Protocol

Perhaps the single most successful international agreement to date has been the Montreal Protocol.

(Kofi Annan, Secretary General of the United Nations)

In 1985, the Vienna Convention established mechanisms for international co-operation in research into the ozone layer and the effects of ODS. 1985 also marked the first discovery of the Antarctic ozone hole. On the basis of the Vienna Convention, the Montreal Protocol on Substances that Deplete the Ozone Layer was negotiated and signed by 24 countries and by the European Economic Community in September 1987. The Protocol called for the Parties to phase down the use of CFCs, halons and other man-made ODS.

After a series of rigorous meetings and negotiations, the Montreal Protocol on Substances that Deplete the Ozone Layer was finally agreed upon on 16 September 1987 in Montreal. The Montreal Protocol stipulates that the production and consumption of compounds that deplete ozone in the stratosphere – chlorofluoro-carbons (CFCs), halons, carbon tetrachloride, and methyl chloroform – are to be phased out by 2000.

The Montreal Protocol on Substances that Deplete the Ozone Layer is one of the first international environmental agreements that includes trade sanctions to achieve the stated goals of a treaty. It also offers major incentives for nations to sign the agreement. The treaty negotiators justified the sanctions because depletion of the ozone layer is an environmental problem most effectively addressed on the global level. Furthermore, without the trade sanctions, there would be economic incentives for non-signatories to increase production, damaging the competitive-ness of the industries in the signatory nations as well as decreasing the search for less damaging CFC alternatives.

Additional measures are currently being proposed by the European Commission and others to accelerate the phase out of various ODC and thereby to provide additional protection for the ozone layer (Europa 2005).

The problem of countervailing risks

CFCs are now identified as rogue chemicals with the capability of creating immense harm. But they were not always perceived that way. In fact, in the 1930s, CFCs were seen as wonder chemicals because they were non-toxic, non-flammable, could be used as refrigerants in place of the highly toxic ammonia compounds then in use, and, so far as anyone knew, were inert. Perhaps this error can be excused, for the chemistry of the upper atmosphere was little understood at that time, but there is a lesson which should be acknowledged, and that is that well-meant interventions may have disturbing side-effects. The implication is that interventions should be screened for their potential to cause unexpected harm, just as health care patients should be warned about the side-effects of prescription drugs.

✏ Activity 20.1

Read the following abridged passages from the Government of Alberta and from Jonathan Wiener, and note the concern about possible new (countervailing) risks cre-ated by CFC replacements. Weiner's analysis was published in 1995 and some things have since changed, but the central point here is not the detailed technical content but the existence of risk trade-offs:

1   In the light of this information, what questions should a policy maker ask?
2   The example here is specifically about ozone-depleting compounds but potentially the problem of creating new risks while removing others is much more widespread. Write down a list of six such situations from as wide a range of environmental health areas as your imagination allows.

 Government of Alberta (2004)

CFCs have ideal thermodynamic properties for use as refrigerants. They are non-flammable, chemically stable and low in toxicity. However, the stability of these refrigerants and their chlorine content have linked them to the depletion of the stratospheric ozone layer . . . depletion of which increases the amount of damaging ultraviolet radiation that penetrates to the earth's surface. The net effect will likely be significant increases in skin cancers in humans and dramatic changes in weather patterns.

Hydrofluorocarbons (HFCs) and hydrochlorofluorocarbons (HCFCs) are considered the replacements for CFCs in refrigeration and air conditioning systems. The HFCs do not contain chlorine, for example, and their potential for depleting the ozone layer is signifi-cantly less than that of CFCs. However, while more environmentally-friendly, the CFC substitutes pose different health and safety concerns to users, such as increased toxicity or flammability . . . Animal studies have linked exposure to some of these compounds with liver damage and liver tumour formation.

Jonathan Wiener (1995)

But HCFCs and HFCs pose other problems. First, some of these compounds are toxic, at least to laboratory animals, renewing the original concern that led CFCs to replace ammonia. Second, using HCFCs for refrigeration can be significantly more costly than using CFCs, up to five times the price. This may be a small issue in industrialized countries, but it is a critical issue of public health risk in poorer countries. From the perspective of those countries, the target risk of most vital concern is food spoilage, which afflicts millions of people annually through hunger, malnutrition, and food-borne disease (World Bank 1992). From the perspective of many industrialized nations and environmental groups, the target risk is global ozone depletion, and increased CFC use in developing countries would pose a risk offset – the same risk imposed globally – thus providing these wealthier countries strong incentives to assist developing countries to make the transition to refrigeration without increasing the use of CFCs. Third, switching to HCFCs and HFCs to reduce ozone depletion may pose an increased risk of a different environmental threat: global warming.

 Feedback

The new risks identified are health and safety through, mainly, occupational exposure; implications for food spoilage in developing countries; and possible impacts on global warming.

1 Policy makers are always in a situation which involves trade-offs. Sometimes they are simple and obvious as in the case of investing finite resources for health gains, but very often there are additional unwanted side-effects and these are not necessarily

small. The advice is that all significant interventions should be scrutinized for their likely non-target effects, and these should be assessed so that a full balance sheet of associated gains and losses can be set up before a decision on whether to go ahead is made.

2 The problem of risk trade-offs, the creation of new risks while dealing with old risks, is ubiquitous. A few examples, by way of illustration, include: prohibiting the use of DDT on environmental grounds increases the number of cases of malaria because DDT is cheap and effective and changes the risk to farmers who must use more toxic organophosphate products; removing lead from gasoline results in higher fuel consumption and hence higher emissions of toxic gaseous pollutants; restrictions on the movements of nuclear waste (mainly proposed on ethical grounds) means that nuclear waste is not always dealt with by those best able to do so; the imposition of strict safety standards on children's playgrounds results in many playgrounds being closed; the chlorination of drinking water to combat waterborne microbial disease poses a (small) cancer risk; evacuating people from their homelands because of some environmental hazard greatly increases stress and associated health effects, and deprives them of their heritage; refusal of permission on health grounds to build a waste incinerator may mean it has to be disposed of by landfill. In each case, it should be incumbent on the policy maker to assess the benefits and disbenefits, including costs, prior to deciding what to do.

The phenomenon of risk trade-offs

John Graham and Jonathan Wiener (1995) state that their research finds that risk trade-offs are not an imagined and inevitable perversity of life but rather a real consequence of incomplete decision making, and that with attention and effort, policy makers can wage the campaign to manage environmental health with better tools that help to recognize and progressively reduce overall risk. This, they say, is important because in their view risk trade-offs are seriously hindering campaigns to improve health. Thus, Graham and Wiener propose a framework for systematic 'risk trade-off' analysis which policy makers could apply at any level to environmental health problems.

 Activity 20.2

In reading the following passage adapted from Graham and Wiener (1995) think about:

1 How their approach aligns itself with the concerns expressed by Mary O'Brien in Chapter 16.
2 Identify interventions which give rise to each of the four varieties of risk trade-off shown in Figure 20.1. You could start with those you identified in Activity 20.1, or those listed in the feedback.
3 How does the proposition that risk trade-off analysis amounts to front-loading the policy process tie in with other changes in the approach to environmental policy making which you have read about?

Systematic risk trade-off analysis

The development of a more systematic, rigorous method for recognizing and resolving risk trade-offs begins with the realization that there is no magic recipe. Weighing risk versus risk will often require both objective information and personal judgment, both expert analysis and ethical values. Some countervailing risks may be deemed sufficiently unimportant that it is worth tolerating them; at other times the countervailing risks may rival, or even outweigh, the net benefits from the reduction in the target risk. In many cases the countervailing risks will be important enough to affect the decision – warranting a modification of the intervention so that it addresses the countervailing risks as well as the target risk – but not so grave that addressing the target risk is wholly undesirable.

The method of risk trade-off analysis (RTA) that we have developed attempts to illuminate and characterize risk trade-offs and to aid in their resolution. Our development of RTA begins with a typology of risk trade-offs that helps policy makers recognize the trade-offs that might occur from an intervention. Second, RTA posits a set of factors for decision makers to evaluate in weighing the comparative importance of target risks and countervailing risks when hard choices must be made. Third, RTA analyzes the possibility of overall risk reduction through 'risk superior' moves.

RTA's aim is to examine the ripples made by an intervention not just in the target area but in the broader range of consequences it may affect. These ripples may extend into non-environmental domains and to international effects; the point is to discard the categorical boundaries that constrain current thinking and encompass more of the comprehensive whole. RTA can thus be one tool in the shift toward a more integrated, comprehensive approach to environmental health policy formulation.

Although RTA requires information and therefore itself gives rise to costs, there may well be attractive efficiencies in its use. RTA may not be increasing the total informational and analytic resources required so much as front-loading those resources in analysis accompanying the decision. The more holistic approach taken in RTA may thus help avoid the subsequent conflicts, delays, and course reversals that would occur if countervailing risks were excluded from the initial decision and the victims of those countervailing risks later returned to the table to demand changes in settled policies.

Like all complex phenomena, risk trade-offs are difficult to describe coherently and comprehensively. Figure 20.1 presents a conceptual matrix that has been helpful to us in

	Compared to the target risk, the countervailing risk is:	
	SAME TYPE	DIFFERENT TYPE
Compared to the target risk, the countervailing risk affects: SAME POPULATION	Risk offset	Risk substitution
DIFFERENT POPULATION	Risk transfer	Risk transformation

Figure 20.1 Typology of risk trade-offs

Source: Graham and Wiener (1995)

describing the phenomenon. Here, the term 'target risk' refers to the risk that is the primary focus of the policy whereas the 'countervailing' risk is the chance of an adverse outcome that results from the attempt to reduce the target risk.

Feedback

1 Though Graham and Wiener have a different approach and possibly a different philosophy, you will observe that their message shares common ground with that of Mary O'Brien whose strong concern was that the scope of risk assessment needed to be broader and more flexible, in order to allow consideration of non-target risks and alternatives.

2 Regarding the activities listed in the feedback: the DDT example is one of risk transformation because different people are affected in new ways; lead removal from petrol is a risk offset because one pollutant is replaced by others; restrictions on nuclear waste movements mean that different people bear the burden of the same risk and constitutes a risk transfer; the children's playground example is one of risk substitution because children are protected from injury but have less opportunity for exercise leading to reduced health; the chlorination example is one of risk offset; and the case of evacuation affects the same population but in very different ways and so is a risk substitution.

3 The proposition fits in well with the trend in thinking towards a more holistic approach to the framing of policy issues. This is illustrated, for example, by Figure 17.1 as compared with Figure 3.2, and by Figure 17.2, as well as ideas brought to bear in Chapters 14 to 16.

Activity 20.3

Given that policy will frequently run into the problem of risk trade-offs, decision makers are going to have to choose between different risk types. On what basis could this be done? What factors should be considered?

Feedback

Policy makers will in most cases be unable to eliminate all countervailing risks. To decide if an intervention is overall beneficial or not, the characteristics of the reduced target risk and the newly created risks must be compared. Obvious parameters for consideration are the magnitude (probability of occurrence) of each risk, the size of population exposed, the type of consequence expected, the reliability of the forecasts, and equity including distributional considerations (who bears each risk). Less obvious is the degree to which qualitative factors of the kind described by Paul Slovic and colleagues in Chapter 12 should influence decisions.

'Risk superior' moves

Graham and Wiener's model of risk trade-offs, with its all-too-obvious grounding in reality, could be seen as disheartening by policy makers. Undoubtedly it imposes a serious challenge, but, as is sometimes correctly recognized, 'Good decisions are hard to make', and no-one ever promised that the environmental health policy makers lot was going to be an easy one, why else would Sarah Lichtenstein and colleagues (Chapter 18) express their compassion for them? On a more optimistic note, Graham and Wiener have this to say:

we believe that contemporary social systems leave room for improvement and that, with intelligent efforts, superior choices can be found through which overall risk can decline. 'Risk reduction' is thus a meaningful goal: choices can be made that on balance, make the world safer for humans and other life forms.

Why are risk trade-offs overlooked?

Just as 'market failures' occur when markets fail to maximize social well-being because the full set of consequences is not considered by market decision makers, so may risk trade-offs occur if policy makers fail to take proper account of the externalities which derive from their interventions. But why does this happen? Why are decisions made without due reflection on the full range of impacts? Graham and Wiener (1995) offer the following suggestions:

Omitted voices

This refers to the absence of some affected parties from the decision process who may have particular interests at stake or who may have specific useful knowledge. Or, as cultural theory reminds us, it could be to do with people who hold a particular world-view and which should at least be recognized in the decision process. As you have read, front-end framing of decision processes to include stakeholders and public interest groups is now intended to address this deficiency.

Use of heuristics

You will recall from Chapter 12 that heuristics are simplified mental models that aid decision processes. When policy makers are presented with large bodies of information there is a tendency to focus on the problem of immediate concern, leaving the wider picture for another day. A variant of this is the tendency to focus on events which are salient, especially in the aftermath of some disaster, like a train crash, or an unusual event, such that issues of greater long-term significance are lost from view.

Bounded specialization

A powerful source of risk trade-offs is located in the structures of society and organizations. Many agencies responsible for policy have either been granted very specific remits, or may have structured themselves in such a way as to have created an infrastructure each part of which is circumscribed in what it can consider and do. This 'bounded specialization' phenomenon is deeply rooted in many agencies dealing with human and environmental health. There are obvious benefits associated with such an approach, which is why it is so widespread, for example, the capability to understand specific problems in depth. However, the loss is that decision makers may be 'blind' to risks just outside of their jurisdiction.

Uninformed people

A further explanation which should not be discounted is that people may simply be uninformed or not want to know. The story of methyl bromide, a powerful ozone-depleting chemical used as a pesticide, as recounted by Mary O'Brien, demonstrates how these factors could in that case have led to a preservation of the status quo rather than a full examination of the possibilities.

 Methyl bromide

From 1992 to 1997 I served as a member of the Methyl Bromide Technical Options Committee. This Montreal Protocol Committee was charged with assembling a report on existing and potential alternatives to using the potent, ozone-depleting pesticide, methyl bromide, as a soil fumigant (i.e., to kill all soil organisms with poisonous fumes); structural fumigant (e.g., in ships' holds, granaries, and homes); and fumigant of durable and perishable commodities of international trade such as wood, grains, fruits, vegetables and flowers. In other words, the Committee was charged with conducting an alternatives assessment. Its report would be used to help determine the schedule of a worldwide phaseout of methyl bromide use.

The process of exploring alternatives to methyl bromide within the Committee was eye-opening. Only a small minority was publicly supportive of alternatives, and even fewer knew of non-chemical alternatives to the pesticide. However, the Committee's mandate to discuss all feasible technical options lent clout to the minority of members who did have knowledge of non-chemical alternatives. If a committee member could provide evidence that a particular alternative was in use or close to availability, it had to be entered into the report. The definition of an alternative to methyl bromide adopted by the Committee was also critical: 'A technology demonstrated or in use in one region of the world that would be applicable in another unless there were obvious technical constraints to the contrary.'

Notably, economic considerations were dealt with elsewhere, so it was possible to discuss all options. The resulting picture of alternatives, including non-chemical alternatives, is impressive. The Committee revealed that technically, alternatives already existed for 90% by volume of worldwide methyl bromide use.

The US Department of Defense, for instance, together with shipping companies and the University of California at Davis, has been successful in developing an alternative to one use of methyl bromide. Prior to 1994, the DoD had been shipping fresh produce by air to US military personnel stationed overseas. The produce was fumigated with methyl bromide to quickly kill insects or mites prohibited in the country to which the produce was being shipped.

The alternative the DoD developed is 'controlled atmosphere' technology in refrigerated vans. This uses optimum combinations and concentrations of nitrogen, carbon dioxide, and oxygen to retain freshness of perishable commodities and to eliminate or prevent the presence of quarantined organisms. The produce is treated during shipment by sea, but arrives in better condition than when fumigated and flown. The DoD is saving millions of dollars. The technique is also applicable to many fruits and vegetables traded between countries.

Many Committee members resisted reporting the existence of alternatives. Those members were invested one way or another (either economically or in a government agency supportive of methyl bromide-using industries) in continuing the use of methyl bromide. If the Committee had not had such a clear mandate and definition of 'alternative', the report would have claimed that continued methyl bromide use was essential.

Public reporting of the existence of alternatives (as in the case of methyl bromide) *is* a powerful process. It can be extremely threatening to the status quo.

Factors affecting policy implementation

While concern about the ozone layer and greenhouse gas accumulation in the atmosphere, fed by scientific research, is growing, there remains a further highly problematic stage prior to the necessary global-scale action being taken. This is the negotiation of international agreements which are binding and effective.

 Activity 20.4

The following passage adapted from an article by Joseph Bial and colleagues (2000) describes factors that influence the translation of environmental concerns into policies and international treaties. The example used here, which exhibits the full range of factors, is the accumulation of greenhouse gases in the atmosphere. In reading the extract make notes on the following:

1   What do you understand by 'an open-access resource problem'?
2   Why is it so difficult to negotiate international agreements on global environmental problems?
3   Under what circumstances is it easier to reach agreement over collective action?

 Translation of environmental concerns into policies

Concerns about the accumulation of greenhouse gases in the atmosphere and possible effects on global temperatures have led to a series of international initiates for collective action. These include the UN Framework Convention on Climate Change (FCCC) signed at Rio de Janeiro in 1992 where countries pledged to voluntarily reduce carbon emissions to 1990 levels by 2000; a meeting in 1995 in Berlin of the Conference of Parties (COP), created at the Rio conference, to define a structure for further action; and the Kyoto Protocol on Global Warming of December 1997.

Global warming is an open-access resource problem. With access to the atmosphere unrestricted, gases such as carbon dioxide (CO_2), nitrous oxide, CFCs and methane are released as by-products of human activities and other natural sources across countries. CFCs are the most potent per molecule, but CO_2 is the most abundant. Regardless of their origin the gases are spread around the globe with potential external effects. The gases retard the re-radiation of the sun's energy from the earth's surface back into space. Under debate are whether and how much the further accumulation of these gases from human actions will generate a damaging rise in global temperatures. The causal relationship between the build-up of greenhouse gases and an increase in global temperatures has not been defined conclusively and hence is subject to debate. Nevertheless, the expected linkages have stimulated international efforts to control emissions and thereby mitigate any possible rise in temperatures.

Most of the focus has been on CO_2, which is released from burning fossil fuels, such as coal, and the USA is currently the largest emitter. At least some restructuring of the American and other industrial economies likely will be necessary with a possible reduction in gross domestic product (GDP). The macroeconomic effects, however, are uncertain because they depend on each country's energy intensity of production, energy sources, and the magnitude and pace of emission reductions implemented. On a microeconomic level, there will be important distributional effects within and across countries, both from global warming and from regulation. Some countries appear to be more vulnerable to any negative implications of global warming and within countries, energy-intensive industries are apt to bear the brunt of emission controls. Taxpayers may be called on to fund the implementation and monitoring of regulations, and to pay for compensating transfers to sectors harmed. Further, they may be required to pay for side payments to other countries as inducements to participate in collective action. These heterogeneous constituent effects and the uncertainty confronted by each party in calculating the net effects of the treaty create political problems for politicians with implications for the success of international collective action.

Effective collective action to address potential climate change will be a formidable challenge. The very nature of global environmental externalities presents incentive problems. Abatement by any country benefits others as a public good, but if abatement is costly to a country's citizens, its politicians have incentive to invest less in reduction efforts than would be globally optimal and free ride on cutbacks taken elsewhere. Research on collective action to address more tractable, local common-property resources indicates that these incentive problems can occur even when there is agreement about the magnitude of the problem and the aggregate benefits of resolving it. These bargaining issues are more complex in international environmental agreements where the benefits and costs are very uncertain and differentially spread across and within countries, and where compliance is voluntary.

Nor do international negotiations take place detached from the underlying political realities within each of the bargaining countries. Rather, a country is represented by an agent who is accountable to domestic constituencies. This agent must adopt an international negotiating position that simultaneously leads to a resolution of the international common-property problem *and* generates the greatest political support among his/her electorate. Thus, the benefits and costs of an international treaty are borne not only by the underlying constituencies, but also by the elected agent. Hence, the agent will be very cautious before committing his/her country to an agreement because imposing even minor costs on a constituency without commensurate benefits may lead to large defections in political support. The political problem faced by politicians is exacerbated if there is considerable uncertainty in estimating constituent benefits and costs from international action.

To summarize, the potential benefits of reduced emissions require coordinated inter-national actions but will be apparent only well into the future. Consequently, no single polluting party will observe any short-term private gain from reducing fossil fuel use. In the absence of clear payoffs for individual actions, politicians in all participating countries face the task of convincing their constituencies of the public good involved in adhering to CO_2 reductions. The political will for these actions, however, will deteriorate if the local costs of regulation are high within a country and there are important uncertainties as to the linkage between current emissions and global temperatures and the magnitude of the costs (or benefits) of a warmer planet.

 Feedback

1 This refers to a resource which is freely available for everyone to use, and sometimes referred to as 'the tragedy of the commons'.

2 International treaties to control environmental pollution have macroeconomic effects on countries which will affect their GDP, and microeconomic effects which raise distribution of wealth issues both within and between countries. Some of these issues can be dealt with by transfer payments, but these are hard to negotiate especially where the impacts of agreements are uncertain. Furthermore, politicians who negotiate such agreements are likely to be very cautious about agreeing anything which will be seen to have an undesirable effect on their constituencies. In the case of global environmental issues like greenhouse gas warming, and to a lesser extent the ozone layer, there is no short-term gain but a high up-front cost. Such 'deals' are usually regarded as unfavourable.

3 Collective agreements could be expected to be simpler to conclude in situations where there is a consensus about the aggregate benefit of some intervention; the parties all perceive positive net gains for their constituency from the agreement; the parties have common bargaining objectives; there are no large distributional issues. Agreements under these conditions tend to be easier because it is in the interest of all parties. In situations where distributional issues arise, these may be resolvable by transfer payments, but this is only likely if the aggregate benefit of the international agreement is positive.

Summary

Environmental health issues at the global level present policy makers with their most formidable challenge. On the one hand, interventions on this scale will inevitably prompt effects which are unintended and undesired, as well as bringing about the benefits sought. Policy makers will need to take a very broad perspective when contemplating interventions on this scale, and must expect to be in a pos-ition of weighing up the advantages and disadvantages of alternative policies. Nonetheless, there will be many situations in which policy makers will find themselves constrained, or in situations in which other parties will want to take a narrower view. In most circumstances, this tendency should be resisted. The nego-tiation of international agreements to implement policy should be expected to be particularly demanding given that there will be imperatives on both the domestic and the international fronts which will in many cases be difficult to reconcile.

References

Bial JJ, Houser D and Libecap GD (2000) *Public choice issues in international collective action: global warming regulation.* http://citeseer.ist.psu.edu/bial00public.html

Europa (2005) *The Ozone Layer.* Available at: http://www.europa.eu.int/comm/environment/ozone/ozone_layer.htm

Government of Alberta (2004) *Health and Safety Issues Associated with the Refrigerant HCFC-123.* Edmonton: Government of Alberta.

Graham JD and Wiener JB (1995) *Risk Versus Risk: Tradeoffs in Protecting Health and the Environment.* Cambridge, MA: Harvard University Press.

O'Brien M (2000) *Making Better Environmental Decisions: An Alternative to Risk Assessment.* Cambridge, MA: MIT Press.

Slovic P, Fischhoff B and Lichtenstein S (1980) Facts and fears: understanding perceived risk, in Schwing RC and Albers WA, *Societal Risk Assessment: How Safe Is Safe Enough?* New York: Plenum.

Wiener JB (2005) Protecting the global environment, in Graham JD and Wiener JB *Risk Versus Risk: Tradeoffs in Protecting Health and the Environment.* Cambridge, MA: Harvard University Press.

World Bank (1992) *World Development Report: Environment and Development.* Washington, DC: World Bank.

Glossary

α value The monetary value of the man-sievert.

Acceptable daily intake (ADI) The daily intake of a chemical which, during a lifetime, appears to be without appreciable risk. Usually measured in mg/kg/day.

Acute exposure A short exposure, typically of hours or minutes, possibly at a high level.

Affect The automatic feeling of goodness or badness generated in response to some event.

Agenda 21 A global plan led by the United Nations which seeks to integrate environmental, social and health issues into decision making.

Alternatives assessment A process that involves looking at the risks, benefits and other pros and cons of a broad range of environmental health policy options.

Analytic-deliberation A process of decision making which involves both technical analysis and engagement with affected and interested parties.

As low as reasonably achievable (ALARA) A fundamental concept in radiological protection, sometimes known as 'optimization'.

As low as reasonably practicable (ALARP) In some countries a fundamental concept in safety assessment.

Best available technique not entailing excessive cost (BATNEEC) A pollution control philosophy.

Best practicable environmental option (BPEO) A pollution control philosophy.

Bioaccumulation A process which results in the concentration of particular substances being higher in some organisms than in their surrounding environment.

Capacity 21 and 2015 Capacity-building programmes that support Agenda 21 and the quest for sustainability.

Carcinogen Any chemical or physical agent able to induce cancer in living organisms.

Carcinogenesis The process of the origination, causation and development of malignant tumours.

Case-control study An observational study starting with the identification of a group of cases and controls. The level of exposure to the risk factor of interest can then be measured (retrospectively) and compared.

Chronic exposure An exposure of long duration, months or years, and usually to a low concentration.

Cohort A group or population that share a common characteristic.

Cohort study A follow-up observational study where groups of individuals are defined on the basis of their exposure to a certain suspected risk factor for a disease.

Collective dose The sum of the radiation doses to the individuals within a specified group, measured in units called man-sieverts.

Communitarianism A philosophy that values communities and resists the idea that individuals and free market exchanges are the key social institutions.

Confounding variable (confounder) A variable that is associated with the exposure under study and is also a risk factor for the outcome in its own right.

Conservatism Assuming a worst case scenario in order to err on the side of safety.

Contingent valuation Survey approach to asking individuals to imagine markets exist and to give their willingness to pay for (accept) benefits (losses).

Countervailing risk A newly created risk that results from action to reduce a target risk.

Cross-sectional study A study design where exposure and outcome are measured at the same time.

Cultural theory A social theory that proposes that social responses to risks are determined by cultural belief patterns and not objective facts about risk.

Deliberation A reciprocal exchange of ideas between the public, interest groups and policy makers.

de manifestis When applied to risk, refers to levels which are manifestly intolerable.

de minimis When applied to risk, refers to levels which are considered trivial or negligible.

Deoxyribonucleic acid (DNA) The molecule in which the genetic blueprint for living cells is encoded.

Deterministic effects Effects which can be directly associated with their causes and which generally increase as dose increases. Normally a threshold exists.

Dose A stated quantity or concentration of a substance to which an organism is exposed over either a continuous or an intermittent period. Dose is most commonly measured in units of milligrams per kilogram of body weight of the receiver (mg/kg bw).

Dose equivalent A measure of the amount of radiation absorbed by tissue combined with a factor accounting for the ability of the type of radiation involved to cause damage, measured in units called sieverts.

Dose limit The officially recognized maximum tolerable dose of ionizing radiation during a specified time interval.

Dose–response assessment The determination of the relationship between administered doses and the incidence or severity of the associated adverse effects.

Ecological fallacy The effects measured in groups may not be applicable at the level of individuals.

Effective dose equivalent The dose equivalent incorporating a further weighting to account for the vulnerability to harm of the body part exposed, measured in units called sieverts.

Egalitarianism A moral perspective emphasizing equality of people.

Environmental agent Any chemical, biological or physical substance, or social factor, which is under investigation.

Environmental health Those aspects of human health and disease that are determined by factors in the environment.

Environmental impact assessment A technique and process by which information about the environmental effects of a project is collected.

Environmental medium A specific part of the environment such as air, water or soil, sometimes referred to as an environmental compartment.

Epidemiology The study of the distribution and determinants of health states or events in specified populations, and the application of this study to the control of health problems.

Ex-ante decisions Decisions that are made in advance of some potential outcome.

Experiential learning Learning from experience.

Exposure The degree to which a person is subject to a given risk factor.

Exposure assessment A qualitative or quantitative estimation of the magnitude, frequency and duration of exposure of the general population, sub-groups or individuals, to hazardous substances or situations.

Exposure pathway The means by which risk agents come into contact with target organisms, e.g. via drinking water, inhalation, dermal contact, or physical proximity, etc.

Exposure route How an agent enters the body (such as by inhalation, ingestion, contact).

Expressed preference studies Studies that elicit consumers' preferences by asking them questions about real or hypothetical scenarios.

Externality Cost or benefit arising from an individual's production or consumption decision which indirectly affects the well-being of others.

Genotoxic A chemical that can cause damage in genetic material leading to heritable changes.

Governance The process of governing, or of controlling, managing, or regulating the affairs of some entity.

Hazard A factor or exposure that may adversely affect health.

Hazard identification The identification of adverse health or environmental effects which could be associated with an agent or situation should exposure arise.

Hazard index (HI) The quotient of the maximum daily dose and the acceptable daily intake of an hazardous material.

Health impact assessment A method which aims to identify the likely changes in health risk of a policy, programme, plan, or development action on a defined population.

Human exposure – rodent potency index (HERP) An index devised for ranking the risk of potential human carcinogens based on average human exposure and rodent toxicity data.

Incidence The frequency of new cases in a defined population during a specified period of time.

in vitro A laboratory test using living cells taken from an organism.

in vivo A laboratory test carried out on living organisms such as whole animals or human volunteers.

Ionizing radiation Radiation that is sufficiently energetic to break the bonds that hold molecules together to form ions.

LD$_{50}$ The dose that when administered to animals in a test is lethal to 50 per cent.

Linear no threshold hypothesis The presumption that risk is linearly related to dose at low doses for non-threshold agents.

Lowest observed adverse effect level The lowest experimental or observed concentration or amount of a substance that causes adverse alterations in target organisms.

Multi-hit model Dose–response models that assume that more than one interaction with a toxic material at the molecular level is necessary to cause an effect.

Mutagen An agent which can cause genetic damage to individual cells.

No observed adverse effect level (NOAEL) The highest dose at which no significant adverse effects are noticed in a population.

Objectivism The idea that risks can be measured and that we can distinguish between their real magnitude and what people variously and perhaps erroneously believe them to be.

One-hit model Dose–response models that assume that a response occurs after a target has been impacted once at the molecular level by a biologically effective dose.

Opportunity (economic) cost The value of the next best alternative foregone as a result of the decision made.

Pareto rule An intervention satisfying this rule would improve the well-being of some people without harming anyone else.

Policy Broad statement of goals, objectives and means that create the framework for activity. Often take the form of explicit written documents but may also be implicit or unwritten.

Potential Pareto improvement (Kaldor–Hicks principle) The basis for cost–benefit analysis. It stipulates that a reallocation of resources which makes someone better off and someone worse off represents an improvement only as long as those who gain could potentially compensate those who lose.

Precautionary principle A principle that advocates the use of prudent social policy in the absence of empirical evidence in an attempt to solve a problem.

Prevalence The frequency of existing cases in a defined population at a particular point in time (point prevalence), or over a given period of time (period prevalence), as a proportion of the total population.

Probability A quantitative or qualitative expression of the likelihood or chance that a particular outcome will occur as a result of a specified cause or action.

Psychometric paradigm An approach to understanding public attitudes to different risks based on the use of quantitative techniques.

Psychometrics The science of psychological measurement.

Quality-adjusted life year (QALY) A year of life adjusted for its quality of its value. A year in perfect health is considered equal to 1.0 QALY.

Rational actor paradigm (RAP) A sociological theory of human behaviour based on people acting as self-seeking individuals and maximizing their personal utility.

Reference dose An estimate of the highest daily dosage of a risk agent that is unlikely to produce an appreciable harmful effect in humans.

Relativism An extreme doctrine in which anyone's opinion is as good as anyone else's.

Revealed preference studies Studies of actual consumer behaviour which indirectly reveal their preferences.

Risk The probability that an event will occur within a specified time.

Risk assessment A method for estimating the probability or likelihood of a specified type of harm occurring to an individual or a population.

Risk aversion The unwillingness of an individual to take on an identified risk.

Risk-based thinking An approach to decision making that relies in part upon risk assessment.

Risk characterization A synthesis and summary of information about a potentially hazardous situation that addresses the needs and interests of decision makers and of interested and affected parties. Risk characterization is a prelude to decision making and depends on an iterative, analytic-deliberative process.

Risk communication Any meaningful communication between parties over matters of risk; not restricted simply to one-way communication.

Risk governance Encompasses the totality of participants, rules, conventions, processes and mechanisms concerned with the collection, analysis and communication of relevant information, and the making of policy decisions.

Risk management The use of risk assessment in combination with socio-economic and political inputs to evaluate and select measures to manage risk.

Risk trade-off The change in the portfolio of risks that occurs when a new risk is generated (knowingly or inadvertently) by an intervention to reduce a target risk.

Risk trade-off analysis An organized approach to identifying countervailing risks and assessing the balance of the full risk portfolio associated with a policy intervention.

Safety factor A single factor or several factors used to derive an acceptable intake of a chemical.

Sievert (Sv) A unit of equivalent dose of radiation which relates the absorbed dose in human tissue to the effective biological damage of the radiation. A millisievert (mSv) is one-thousandth of a sievert.

Social capital The institutions, relationships, and norms that shape the quality and quantity of a society's social interactions.

Social constructivism This approach to knowledge denies the existence of reality prior to human engagement and the validity of 'truth' in the sense of a corresponding representation of reality. Instead, it poses that reality is whatever is known, and that all knowledge is socially produced. Constructivism can thus lead to relativism, as it allows no distinction between true and untrue statements.

Social impact assessment The process of assessing or estimating, in advance, the social consequences that are likely to follow from specific policy actions or project developments.

Stakeholder An individual or group with a substantive interest in an issue (i.e. interest group), including those with some role in making a decision or its execution.

Stochastic A random statistical phenomenon.

Stochastic effects Effects that are governed by the laws of probability. The severity of harm is independent of dose, but the probability of experiencing the harm is proportional to the dose. There is no threshold dose below which effects do not occur.

Strategic environmental assessment The formalized, systematic and comprehensive process of evaluating the environmental effects of a policy, plan or programme and its alternatives.

Sustainability Development which meets the needs of the present without compromising the ability of future generations to meet their own needs.

Target risks The risk that is the primary focus of an environmental health intervention.

Teratogen An agent which can induce congenital anomalies in a developing foetus.

Threshold The lowest dose or exposure level which will produce a toxic effect.

Toxicology The study of the adverse effects of chemicals on living organisms.

Unit cancer risk (UCR) An estimate of the excess probability of cancer per unit dose.

Utilitarianism (welfarism) Based on the notion that society's interests are best served through the maximization of individual utilities.

Value of a Statistical Life (VSL) A monetary value used for assessing the efficiency of interventions to improve health or safety of unknown individuals.

Willingness-to-pay (WTP) A method of measuring the value an individual places on reducing the risk of developing a health problem or gaining an improvement in health.

Index

Locators shown in *italics* refer to figures and tables.